SpringerBriefs in Population Studies

Population Studies of Japan

For further volumes:
http://www.springer.com/series/13101

The world population is expected to expand by 39.4 % to 9.6 billion in 2060 (UN World Population Prospects, revised 2010). Meanwhile, Japan is expected to see its population contract by nearly one-third to 86.7 million, and its proportion of the elderly (65 years of age and over) will account for no less than 39.9 % (National Institute of Population and Social Security Research in Japan, Population Projections for Japan 2012). Japan has entered the post-demographic transitional phase and will be the fastest shrinking country in the world, followed by former Eastern bloc nations, leading other Asian countries that are experiencing drastic changes.

A declining population that is rapidly aging impacts a country's economic growth, labor market, pensions, taxation, health care, and housing. The social structure and geographical distribution in the country will drastically change, and short-term as well as long-term solutions for economic and social consequences of this trend will be required.

This series aims to draw attention to Japan's entering the post-demographic transition phase and to present cutting-edge research in Japanese population studies. It will include compact monographs under the editorial supervision of the Population Association of Japan (PAJ).

The PAJ was established in 1948 and organizes researchers with a wide range of interests in population studies of Japan. The major fields are (1) population structure and aging; (2) migration, urbanization, and distribution; (3) fertility; (4) mortality and morbidity; (5) nuptiality, family, and households; (6) labor force and unemployment; (7) population projection and population policy (including family planning); and (8) historical demography. Since 1978, the PAJ has been publishing the academic journal *Jinkogaku Kenkyu* (The Journal of Population Studies), in which most of the articles are written in Japanese.

Thus, the scope of this series spans the entire field of population issues in Japan, impacts on socioeconomic change, and implications for policy measures. It includes population aging, fertility and family formation, household structures, population health, mortality, human geography and regional population, and comparative studies with other countries.

This series will be of great interest to a wide range of researchers in other countries confronting a post-demographic transition stage, demographers, population geographers, sociologists, economists, political scientists, health researchers, and practitioners across a broad spectrum of social sciences.

Toru Suzuki

Low Fertility and Population Aging in Japan and Eastern Asia

Springer

Toru Suzuki
Population Structure Research
National Institute of Population and Social
Security Research
Chiyoda-ku, Tokyo
Japan

ISSN 2198-2724 ISSN 2198-2732 (electronic)
ISBN 978-4-431-54779-2 ISBN 978-4-431-54780-8 (eBook)
DOI 10.1007/978-4-431-54780-8
Springer Tokyo Heidelberg New York Dordrecht London

Library of Congress Control Number: 2013957712

Printed on acid-free paper

Springer is part of Springer Science+Business Media (www.springer.com)

Acknowledgments

The ideas and findings included in this book have gradually developed through my works in a series of research projects on Eastern Asian countries, granted by the Ministry of Health, Labour and Welfare of Japan. Prof. Hiroshi Kojima (Waseda University) originally launched the project and worked as the principal researcher in the first round (2002–2004). I succeeded the position at the second round (2006–2008), and we extend the topics from low fertility to various family changes, working patterns, and population aging. This book was written when we were in the middle of the fourth round (2012–2014). I owe much to Prof. Shoichi Ito (Kwansei Gakuin University), Prof. Naoko Soma (Yokohama National University), and Mr. Keita Suga (National Institute of Population and Social Security Research) who have been working as project members, as well as to Prof. Kojima. Although there are too many names to list up here, I also would like to thank all the researchers in Japan, Korea, Taiwan, China, and other countries, for contributing to and stimulating our projects.

Contents

Low Fertility and Population Aging in Japan and Eastern Asia

1 Introduction: The Plan of the Book

This book compares low fertility and population aging of Japan with those of Eastern Asian countries including the Republic of Korea ("Korea" hereafter), the Republic of China ("Taiwan" hereafter) and the People's Republic of China ("China" hereafter). Korea recorded a Total Fertility Rate (TFR) of 1.08 in 2005, and Taiwan 0.895 in 2010. While these are astonishing figures rarely observed in other parts of the world, Japan's low record TFR of 1.26 in 2005 was around the average of Southern/Eastern European countries that had experienced lowest-low fertility (Kohler et al. 2002) in the 1990s. Patterns of fertility decline and their covariates in Japan, Korea, and Taiwan are examined in Sect. 2. Demographic analysis on "tempo distortion" and decomposition into nuptiality and marital fertility are followed by an examination of proximate determinants and socio-economic factors, including demand for children, the cost of childrearing, labor market condition, and female labor force participation.

There is a cultural divide between moderately low fertility in Northern/Western Europe and English-speaking developed countries and very low fertility in Southern/Eastern Europe, German-speaking countries, and Eastern Asian advanced countries (McDonald 2005, 2009). Demographers have attempted classification of cultural zones in terms of marriage patterns (Hajnal 1965), household formation systems (Hajnal 1982), below-replacement fertility (van de Kaa 1987), and family ties (Reher 1998). The contrast between average lowest-low fertility in Japan (1.26) and extreme lowest-low fertility in Korea (1.08) and Taiwan (0.895) can be seen as another cultural divide. Section 3 contrasts Japan as the offspring of a feudal family with other Eastern Asian countries as the offspring of a Confucian family. Since Western European societies have been at the vanguard of both industrialization and post-industrialization, especially Anglo-Saxon societies, families in such societies are thought to be the most adaptive and have the most advantages with respect to the postindustrial phase of socioeconomic change. It could be said that the more distant the family pattern is from that seen in Northern-Western Europe, the lower the TFR becomes. It is assumed that some

T. Suzuki, *Low Fertility and Population Aging in Japan and Eastern Asia*,
SpringerBriefs in Population Studies of Japan, DOI: 10.1007/978-4-431-54780-8_1,

characteristics of Japan, which shares with Europe a common tradition of feudalism, has resulted in approximately the same level of low fertility as that seen in Southern/Eastern Europe, while the TFR values of Korea and Taiwan have dropped to even lower levels because their family patterns are more distant from Northern/Western European pattern.

China's situation is difficult to determine. Although the country's official TFR of 1.18 in the 2010 census is supposedly unrealistically low, its fertility has been below-replacement level for more than two decades (UNPD 2013). In spite of drastic population aging as expected, the Chinese government has continued to enforce its rigid anti-natal policy. Section 4 discusses policy changes among those Eastern Asian countries that are suffering from low fertility. The Japanese government was shocked with the historically low TFR of 1.57 in 1989, and started to institute pro-natal policy interventions, including those pertaining to child allowance, childcare leave, improvements in daycare services, and a work-life balance campaign. It was after their TFR values dropped to lowest-low level of 1.3 or less that Korea and Taiwan decided to introduce pro-natal policy measures. It seems that a Malthusian nightmare caused by population density higher than Japan, together with an enthusiastic governmental anti-natal campaign that lasted for decades, made political transition difficult. In the case of China, the fear of overpopulation is so serious that it seems impossible to transit to a pro-natal policy before the population actually starts to decline.

Demographically, two sources of population aging are increased longevity and a decline in the population growth rate (Lee 1994). The effect of fertility decline is quite straightforward: it always promotes population aging via declines in growth rate. On the other hand, while a decline in mortality promotes population aging through the individual aging effect, it discourages aging because lower mortality implies a higher growth rate. Thus, the primary cause of population aging is fertility decline; mortality decline has a secondary impact. This does not mean, however, that the impact of mortality is negligible. Japan is presently the most aged country in the world because it has the lowest mortality rate and also a fertility rate as low as that seen in other developed countries. The lower fertility rates of Korea and Taiwan imply that population aging will eventually be more severe there than in Japan. In fact, the UNPD (2013) predicts that measures of population aging in each of Korea and Taiwan will exceed that of Japan around 2060.

It is assumed that the Eastern Asian "miracle" of economic development was supported by the so-called demographic bonus, namely a decline in the total dependency ratio caused by a fertility decline (Mason 2001). However, the impact of a fertility decline on that demographic bonus is less clear because it is outside the range of stable population theory. Section 5 presents a stylized linear model of population aging to examine not only the percentage of the elderly and the median age, but also the dependency ratio and the timing of population decline. The difference between Japan and other Eastern Asian countries in various aspects of population aging will be interpreted from the model.

Because of Eastern Asia's rapid fertility decline, that region's population aging has arrived at an earlier stage of socioeconomic development than was the case in

Japan and other developed countries. It was in 1999 that a universal pension system was established in Korea; in Taiwan it occurred in 2008. China launched a pension system in its rural areas in 2009. In comparison to Japan, which initiated a public pension system in 1961, the provision of support for the elderly in these countries has been difficult. Section 6 examines the politics of population aging in Japan and other Eastern Asian societies. Governments may want to preserve traditional family values to cope with rapid population aging. However, a drastic fertility decline also implies a drastic decline in family resources that can be allocated to the elderly. Thus, this section examines the changing living arrangements among elderly people in Japan and Eastern Asia. It is found that the situation in Korea is more serious than in Taiwan, due to its more compressed urbanization. On the other hand, policy intervention is more advanced in Korea than in Taiwan, especially in terms of a universal pension system. Finally, China's enactment of its Law on the Protection of the Rights and Interests of the Elderly indicates that the government intends to emphasize traditional family values in order to compensate for the slow development of its social security programs.

2 Demography of Low Fertility in Japan and Eastern Asia

2.1 Introduction

When below-replacement fertility emerged in Northern/Western Europe in the 1980s, the second demographic transition theory (van de Kaa 1987) interpreted the trend as a symptom of a value-change syndrome from familism to individualism, along with an increase in cohabitation, extramarital births, divorce, female labor force participation, and living alone. In the 1990s, however, among Southern/ Eastern European countries the TFR dropped to "lowest-low" level of 1.3 or less (Kohler et al. 2002). The emergence of lowest-low fertility drastically changed the correlation between fertility level and family variables. Today, countries with robust marriage institutions, traditional gender roles and strong familism tend to show lower fertility.

Even when the Southern/Eastern European countries in the 1990s experienced historically low fertility levels of less than 1.3, demographers could not have imagined that Eastern Asian advanced countries would eventually be at the forefront of fertility decline. While it is regrettable that no demographic theory could predict this development, we still need to seek interpretations of such an emergent change.

This section examines fertility decline in Japan, Korea and Taiwan. Demographic analysis will be used to examine the effects of delayed childbirth, nuptiality decline, and other proximate determinants. The effects of desired family size, the direct cost of children, economic recession, and female labor force participation are also considered. A more comparative assessment in terms of cultural similarities and differences will be presented in the subsequent sections.

2.2 Unexpected Fertility Decline in Eastern Asia

Demographers have been failing to anticipate emergent changes in fertility. The prediction of classic demographic transition theory that fertility will fluctuate at around the replacement level was rejected with the postwar baby boom and the subsequent spread of below-replacement fertility. The cyclical change asserted by Easterlin (1978) was denied when it became apparent that most developed countries would not regain replacement levels for many generations. When Scandinavian and German-speaking countries led fertility decline into the below-replacement level, the second demographic transition theory (van de Kaa 1987) asserted that the trend was the result of a value change toward individualism and secularization. The theory predicted that fertility decline would proceed together with postmodern family changes (e.g., increases in cohabitation, extramarital births, divorce, female labor force participation, and living alone). The prediction failed due to the emergence of lowest-low fertility, which is defined as a TFR of 1.3 or less (Kohler et al. 2002). A paradoxical situation appeared wherein fertility is lower in countries with more robust marriage institutions, more effective gender segregation, and stronger familism.

In the 2000s, lowest-low fertility started to spread in Eastern Asian advanced countries. Figure 1 shows the development of fertility decline in Japan, Korea, Taiwan, and China, since 1980. While figures for Japan, Korea, and Taiwan are official TFR values published by the government statistical bureaus, official TFR values from Chinese censuses (i.e., 1.22 in 2000 and 1.18 in 2010) are supposedly unrealistically low. Thus, Fig. 1 instead uses TFR values from UNPD (2013).

Although Korea and Taiwan showed TFR values lower than that in Japan in the late 1980s, these countries sustained higher levels than Japan throughout the 1990s. However, the sudden acceleration of fertility decline in Korea and Taiwan following the small millennial baby boom resulted in lower TFR values than that in Japan. Korea arrived at a TFR of 1.3 in 2001, followed by Japan and Taiwan in 2003. While Japan, as well as many European countries, escaped lowest-low fertility after 2005, the TFR values in Korea and Taiwan stayed at the lowest-low level. Korea recorded a TFR of 1.08 in 2005, and that of Taiwan was 0.895 in 2010; the latter is supposedly the record-lowest value for a country with a rural area. Fertility in China seems still be higher than that seen in each of the other three countries. However, the UNPD (2013) assumes that the TFR in China has been at the below-replacement level since the early 1990s.

2.3 Demography of Fertility Decline in Japan

2.3.1 Delay in Childbearing

Most of the advanced industrial countries have shown delays in childbearing; as shown in Fig. 2, those in Eastern Asia are no exception. Korea finished the first fertility transition in the early 1980s, whereupon the mean age at childbirth started

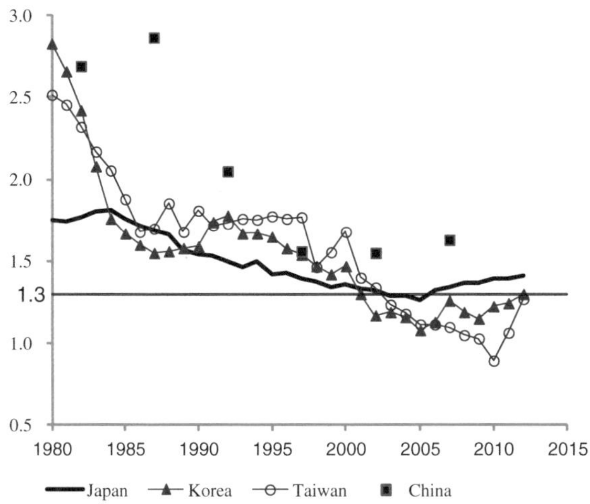

Fig. 1 Total fertility rate in Eastern Asia (UNPD 2013)

Fig. 2 Mean age at childbearing

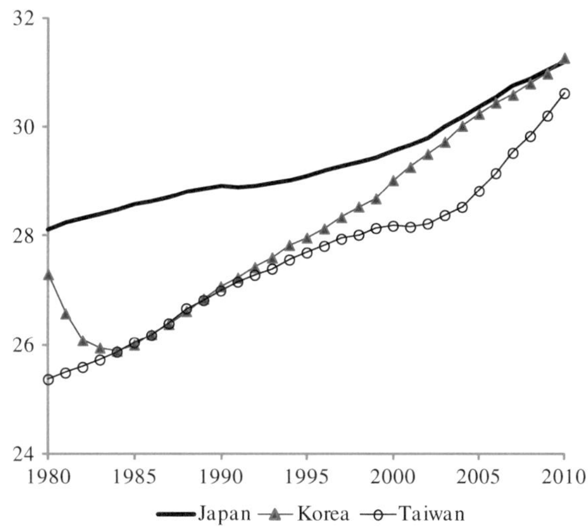

to increase. In Japan and Taiwan, the delay accelerated after 2000. The delay in Korea and Taiwan was faster than Japan. As a result, the mean age at childbearing in 2010 was 31.3 for Korean women, slightly exceeding 31.2 for Japanese women. The mean age among Taiwanese women in 2010 was 30.6 in 2010, but that figure is rapidly catching up with those in Korea and Japan.

It is known that delays in childbirth exaggerate fertility decline as seen through TFR values. Bongaarts and Feeney (1998) formalized how to adjust this tempo distortion. Their Adjusted Total Fertility Rate (ATFR) is defined by birth order:

$$ATFR_i = \frac{TFR_i}{1 - r_i}.$$

Here, r_i is the rate of change in the mean age at childbirth by birth order. In Japan, in the 2000–2010 period, the mean age at all births increased by annual average of 0.16 years. This implies that the TFR of Japan would be higher by 1/ (1 − 0.16) = 19 % if there were no delay in childbirth. In Korea, the annual increase was 0.22 years, which implies that the TFR would be 28 % higher if the delay were to cease immediately. In Taiwan, the annual increase was 0.24 years, which implies that the TFR would be 32 % higher if the delay were to cease immediately. A more accurate magnitude of tempo distortion can be obtained from birth-order specific calculations. However, it suffices here to point out that there has been a considerable exaggeration of fertility decline, and that the magnitude is larger in Korea and Taiwan than in Japan.

2.3.2 Cohort Fertility

The Complete Fertility Rate (CFR) of a real cohort is a measure superior to the TFR, because the latter suffers from both tempo distortion and the parity composition effect. The problem is that the CFR cannot be determined until the cohort completes its reproduction. However, the CFR of cohorts in their forties is predictable, because at this age, only a small number of births will be added to the current level. Figure 3 shows the cumulative fertility relative to that of the 1950 cohort with a CFR of 2.03, using the scheme of Frejka and Calot (2001). Although the 1955 cohort was behind its predecessor in the early twenties, it almost caught up to and fulfilled the CFR of 1.98. However, the decline in CFR for the younger cohort is more significant. The CFR of the 1960 cohort was 1.85. The cumulative fertility of the 1965 cohort was 1.60 at age 46 and the CFR will be approximately the same.

Although it is difficult to predict the CFR of cohorts born after 1970, postponement in the early twenties seems too serious to be compensated for later. Thus, the CFR of younger cohorts in Japan may not arrive at 1.6, which was predicted for Italian cohorts (Frejka and Calot 2001; van Imhoff 2001). The CFR of Japan's 1976–1980 cohort as predicted by d'Addio and Mira d'Ercole (2005) was as low as 1.42. Furthermore, the latest official population projection for Japan (NIPSSR 2012a) assumes that the CFR of the 1975 cohort will be 1.39.

2.3.3 Nuptiality Decline

As Lesthaeghe (2010) mentioned, only one element of the second demographic transition that cannot be found in Eastern Asia is the increase in extramarital births. The percentage of extramarital births shown in the vital statistics of Japan was 2.15 % in 2010, showing very little change from 1.07 % in 1990 and 1.63 % in 2000.

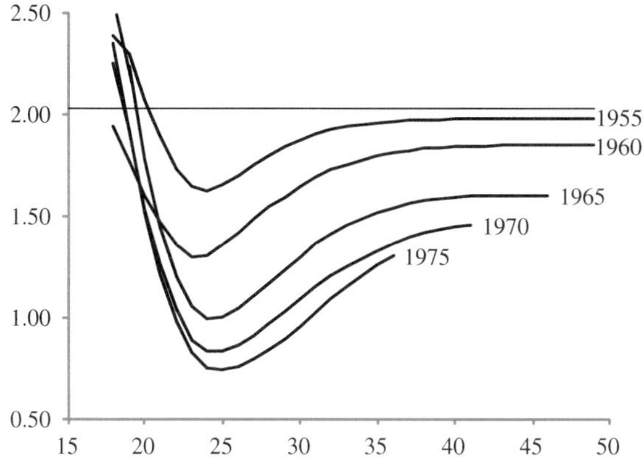

Fig. 3 Cohort fertility compared to 1950 cohort of Japan. NIPSSR (2013)

While Korea shows roughly the same level of extramarital births in 2010 (2.05 %), Taiwan shows a slightly higher proportion in that year (4.51 %). However, the very small percentage of extramarital births in Eastern Asia suggests that the nuptiality decline there has had an important and direct impact on fertility decline.

Nuptiality decline, as with fertility decline, has been more marked in Korea and Taiwan than in Japan. Table 1 compares the percentage of never-married women among three birth cohorts in Japan, Korea and Taiwan. For the cohort born in the early 1970s, Japan showed the highest percentage of never-married women. However, Korean and Taiwanese women quickly caught up with Japanese women in terms of the delay in marriage. In 2010, the percentage of never-married women aged 25–29 (i.e., those born in the early 1980s) was much higher in Korea and Taiwan than in Japan.

As for the role of nuptiality, Japanese demographers asserted until the mid-1990s that nuptiality explains fertility decline in its entity based on Age-specific Marital Fertility Rates (Atoh 1992; Kono 1995; Tsuya and Mason 1995; NIPSSR 1997). However, such results are not reliable, given the serious deficiency inherent in AMFRs (Hirosima 2001; Kaneko 2004).

Let x be the current age, a the age at first marriage, and $y = x - a$ the marital duration. It is assumed that there is no divorce, remarriage, or death during the childbearing age. Thus, the term "marriage" always means first marriage and there is no marital status other than "single" and "(currently) married". The ordinary age-specific fertility rate $f(x)$ can be expressed in terms of marriage rate $n(a)$ and marital fertility rate $m(a, a - x)$ as follows:

$$f(x) = \int_0^x n(a)\, m(a, x - a)\, da, \tag{1}$$

The denominator of an AMFR is the proportion of married women, and it is written as $N(x)$.

Table 1 Proportion never married for female cohorts (%)

Cohort	Country	15–19	20–24	25–29	30–34	35–39
1971–1975	Japan	99.3	86.8	54.0	32.0	23.1
	Korea	99.5	83.3	40.1	19.0	12.6
	Taiwan	–	78.7	47.5	28.7	20.9
1976–1980	Japan	99.3	88.0	59.1	34.5	–
	Korea	99.2	89.1	59.1	29.1	–
	Taiwan	97.8	84.1	61.2	37.2	–
1981–1985	Japan	99.1	88.7	60.3	–	–
	Korea	99.3	93.7	69.3	–	–
	Taiwan	98.4	90.5	70.1	–	–

Based on censuses of Japan and Korea and population register of Taiwan

$$N(x) = \int_0^x n(a)\, da. \tag{2}$$

The AMFR at age x is defined as the ratio of fertility to the proportion married.

$$AMFR(x) = \frac{f(x)}{N(x)} = \frac{\int_0^x n(a)\, m(a, x-a)\, da}{\int_0^x n(a)\, da}. \tag{3}$$

As far as marital fertility is a function of marriage duration, using $N(x)$ as a denominator does not make sense. The ratio is theoretically valid only in the pre-industrial setting, where no intentional birth control is used and marital fertility is a function of age. If $m(a, x - a)$ in (3) is replaced with $m(x)$, then

$$AMFR(x) = \frac{\int_0^x n(a)\, m(x)\, da}{\int_0^x n(a)\, da} = \frac{m(x) \int_0^x n(a)\, da}{\int_0^x n(a)\, da} = m(x). \tag{4}$$

In this case, the age-specific fertility rate is the product of the proportion married and the marital fertility rate. However, when marital fertility is a function of both marriage duration and age at marriage, the ratio is not meaningful.

Decomposition analysis does not necessarily fail, even though AMFRs are not theoretically valid. In the following, ΔTFR is the total change, ΔTFR_n is the change due to marriage behavior, and ΔTFR_m is the change due to childbearing behavior of married couples. It can be seen that age-shift in marriage causes a serious problem that other types of change do not inflict.

$$\Delta TFR = TFR_2 - TFR_1 = \int_0^\infty \{f_2(x) - f_1(x)\}\, dx, \tag{5a}$$

$$\Delta TFR_n = \int_0^\infty \{N_2(x) - N_1(x)\} \cdot \frac{1}{2} \left\{ \frac{f_2(x)}{N_2(x)} + \frac{f_1(x)}{N_1(x)} \right\} dx, \tag{5b}$$

$$\Delta TFR_m = \int_0^\infty \left\{ \frac{f_2(x)}{N_2(x)} - \frac{f_1(x)}{N_1(x)} \right\} \cdot \frac{1}{2} \{N_2(x) + N_1(x)\}\, dx. \tag{5c}$$

Case 1. Age-neutral nuptiality change: Assume that all the age-specific marriage rates are multiplied by a constant *c*. Thus, *n*(*a*) becomes *c n*(*a*). By (1) and (2), the new age-specific fertility rate and the proportion married will be *c f*(*a*) and *c N*(*a*), respectively. Then, there will be no change in age-specific marital fertility rates. The decomposition shows correctly that the nuptiality change caused the fertility change in its entity.

$$\begin{aligned}\Delta TFR_n &= \int_0^\infty \{cN(x) - N(x)\} \cdot \frac{1}{2}\left\{\frac{f(x)}{N(x)} + \frac{f(x)}{N(x)}\right\} dx\\ &= (c-1)\int_\alpha^\beta f(x)dx = TFR_2 - TFR_1,\\ \Delta TFR_m &= \int_0^\infty \left\{\frac{f(x)}{N(x)} - \frac{f(x)}{N(x)}\right\} \cdot \frac{1}{2}\{cN(x) + N(x)\}\, dx = 0.\end{aligned}$$

Case 2. Duration-neutral marital fertility change: Assume that all the marital fertility rates are multiplied by a constant *c*. Thus, *m*(*a,y*) is replaced by *c m*(*a,y*). By (1), the new age-specific fertility rate will be *c f*(*x*). There is no change in the proportion married. Then, the age-specific marital fertility rates will be multiplied by *c*. The decomposition shows correctly that the marital fertility change caused the fertility change in its entity.

$$\begin{aligned}\Delta TFR_n &= \int_0^\infty \{N(x) - N(x)\} \cdot \frac{1}{2}\left\{c\frac{f(x)}{N(x)} + \frac{f(x)}{N(x)}\right\} dx = 0,\\ \Delta TFR_m &= \int_0^\infty \left\{c\frac{f(x)}{N(x)} - \frac{f(x)}{N(x)}\right\} \cdot \frac{1}{2}\{N(x) + N(x)\}\, dx\\ &= (c-1)\int_0^\infty f(x)dx = TFR_2 - TFR_1.\end{aligned}$$

Case 3. Tempo change in marital fertility: Assume that marital fertility rates are uniformly shifted by *h*. Thus, *m*(*a, y*) becomes *m*(*a, y* − *h*) and there is no birth for *h* years after marriage. By (1), the new age-specific fertility rate will also be shifted by *h*. There is no change in the TFR, because the entire fertility schedule is shifted while the quantum remains constant. The decomposition shows correctly that both effects are null.

$$\begin{aligned}\Delta TFR_n &= \int_0^\infty \{N(x) - N(x)\} \cdot \frac{1}{2}\left\{\frac{f(x-h)}{N(x)} + \frac{f(x)}{N(x)}\right\} dx = 0,\\ \Delta TFR_m &= \int_0^\infty \left\{\frac{f(x-h)}{N(x)} - \frac{f(x)}{N(x)}\right\} \cdot \frac{1}{2}\{N(x) + N(x)\}\, dx\\ &= \int_0^\infty f(x-h)dx - \int_0^\infty f(x)dx = 0.\end{aligned}$$

Case 4. Tempo change in marriage: Unfortunately, an age-shift in marriage does not produce such a tidy result, even when the change is an ideal shift without a change in quantum. If we assume that all age-specific marriage rates are uniformly shifted by h, $n(a)$ is replaced by $n(a - h)$. The new age-specific fertility rate and the proportion married are, respectively,

$$f_2(x) = \int_0^x n(a-h)\ m(a, x-a)\, da,$$

$$N_2(x) = \int_0^x n(a-h)\ da = \int_0^{x-h} n(a)\ da = N(x-h).$$

Since there is no change in marital fertility, ΔTFR_m should be zero. However, such a correct result can rarely be obtained. Thus, the use of AMFRs should be avoided whenever there is a change in the timing of marriage.

$$\Delta TFR_m = \frac{1}{2}\Delta TFR + \frac{1}{2}\left\{\int_0^\infty n(a-h)\ M^+(a)\, da - \int_\alpha^{\beta+h} n(a)\ M^-(a)\, da\right\},$$

$$\text{where,} \quad M^+(a) = \int_0^\infty \frac{N(x)}{N(x-h)} m(a, x-a)\, dx,$$

$$M^-(a) = \int_0^\infty \frac{N(x-h)}{N(x)} m(a, x-a)\, dx.$$

More sophisticated methods than those that rely upon the use of AMFRs have shown that nuptiality decline does not explain fertility decline in its entity. Hirosima (1999, 2000) used the proportion of eventually married women and the complete average number of children among married women to decompose the effects of nuptiality and marital fertility. Kaneko (2004) adjusted AMFR by shifting age-specific fertility rates $f(x)$ in accordance with the delay in marriage. Iwasawa (2002) introduced the eventual average number of children by age at marriage to decompose the decline in cohort cumulative fertility. Suzuki (2005) applied the simplified method of Iwasawa to Japan and Korea, assuming that marital fertility does not depend on the age at marriage but solely on the marriage duration. Ogawa (2003) calculated PPPRs (Period Parity Progression Ratios) to decompose fertility decline by parity.

Table 2 summarizes the results of these studies. On the whole, nuptiality decline explains between 35 and 75 % of the TFR decline, depending on the period in question. Thus, it is safe to say that both nuptiality and marital fertility have contributed to the recent fertility decline in Japan, but that their relative importance varies over time.

Unfortunately, Eastern Asian demographers outside of Japan are not aware of the deficit inherent in AMFRs and still rely on the decomposition that makes use of them (Chang 2003; Eun Ki-Soo 2003; Jun 2003; Kim Seung-Kwon 2004c; Lee Sam-Sik 2009; Yap 2009). Some analyses show the apparently erroneous result

Table 2 Contribution of nuptiality in fertility decline in Japan

Literature	Period	Contribution of nuptiality (%)
Hirosima (1999)	1974–1997	40
Hirosima (2000)	1970–2000	70
Iwasawa (2002)	1970–2000	70
Kaneko (2004)	1980–2000	74
Suzuki (2005)	1990–2002	37
Ogawa (2003)	1972–2000	52

that nuptiality explains fertility decline in its entity. Suzuki (2008) attempted a decomposition analysis using a parity progression measure and found that only 31.5 % of fertility decline in 2000–2005 could be attributed to nuptiality decline, while the decline in a second birth explained the largest part. However, as with the case of Japan, the result can be sensitive to the choice of period.

2.3.4 Proximate Determinants

Since marriage does not explain fertility decline in its entity, there should be proximate determinants (Bongaarts 1978) that prompted a significant fall in marital fertility. In Japan, however, neither contraception nor induced abortion constitutes key determinants. According to the Population Problems Research Council (2005), the percentage of currently married women practicing contraception dropped from 55.9 % in 2000 to 52 % in 2004. According to the Report on Public Health Administration and Services (various years), the number of induced abortion in 2010 was 212,694, which is significantly fewer than the 341,146 performed in 2000. The ratio of abortions to live births has also been in decline; it was 14.5 % in 1990, 11.7 % in 2000, and 7.9 % in 2010.

As expected, the frequency of miscarriages has also in decline due to the development in maternal health care program and medical technology. There were 26,560 still births in 2010 in Japan, and their ratio to live births was 2.5 %. This figure is significantly lower than the figures of 4.4 % in 1990 and 3.2 % in 2000. Breastfeeding is not an important proximate determinant in developed countries. Thus, neither intrauterine mortality nor postpartum amenorrhea seems to have contributed to the recent fertility decline in Japan.

The remaining proximate determinants are frequency of intercourse and sterility. There is no time-series data on coital frequency or infecundity among married couples in Japan. It might be possible to assert that the number of sexless couples is increasing due to longer working hours or strengthened mother–child ties. It might also be possible to hypothesize an increase in infecundity due to the rising age at marriage, environmental hormones, and sexually transmitted diseases (Semba 2002). However, it is difficult to evaluate such hypotheses, given the lack of necessary data.

In Korea, the percentage of married women practicing contraception was as high as 79.3 % in 2000, increasing further to 84.5 % in 2003 (Chang Kyung-Sup et al. 2006). This explains a portion of the TFR decline from 1.47 to 1.19 in this period. However, the contraception practice rate declined to 80.2 % in 2005 (Lee Sam-Sik et al. 2005); this event does not correspond to the TFR decline to 1.08. In Taiwan, the percentage of married women who had ever practiced contraception reached 90 % in 1985 (Chu and Yu 2010). Thus, as in Korea, there seems to be little room for change to cause drastic fertility decline in recent decades. Although the trend of induced abortion in Korea or Taiwan is unknown, it is possible that abortion contributed in part to the recent fertility decline. It is unlikely, as in Japan, that still births or breastfeeding have played an important role. If the situation is the same in these two countries as in Japan, the major proximate determinant should be either sexual intercourse or sterility.

2.4 Socioeconomic Determinants

2.4.1 Demands for Children

One important question pertaining to the recent fertility decline is whether it derives from voluntary choice. The low fertility trap hypothesis (Lutz et al. 2006) suggested the possibility of positive feedback between attitude and behavior. The mechanism has already started working in German-speaking countries where the ideal number of children is extremely low. However, very low fertility in Japan and Eastern Asia is not the result of very low demand for children. Figure 4 shows the change in the ideal number of children in three countries. The demand for children in Japan has been declining slowly but was still as high as 2.42 in 2010. In Korea, the ideal number of children was as small as 2.0 in the early 1980s, it gradually recovered to 2.3 in 2005 before declining again in 2010. While married women in Taiwan used to prefer larger families than Japanese and Korean women, in 2003 their preference converged with those in Japan. Although recent data are not available, it seems unlikely that Taiwanese women now have a much smaller preference than Korean women. Thus, it is clear that very low fertility levels in these three countries is not due to low demand for children; rather it should be explained in terms of the obstacles to fulfilling that demand.

2.4.2 Direct Cost of Children

In the world of post-industrialization, globalization and rapid technological innovation, there is a growing demand for human capital investment. Thus, parents are more interested in quality of children, and education costs have become higher (Becker 1991). The rising cost of children, including public and private educational costs, is thought to be a key reason for the recent low fertility rate in Eastern Asia.

Figure 5 shows the trend of college enrollment in three countries. The rise in enrollment in Japan after 1990 was less dramatic than that in either Korea or Taiwan.

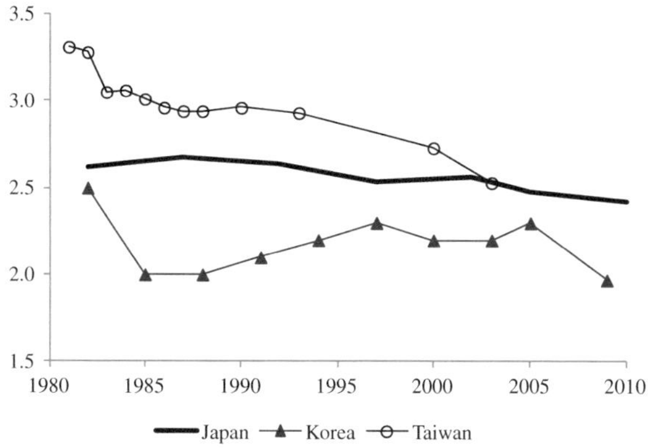

Fig. 4 Ideal number of children for married women. NIPSSR (2012b), Lee Sam-Sik et al. (2005, 2009), DGBAS (2003)

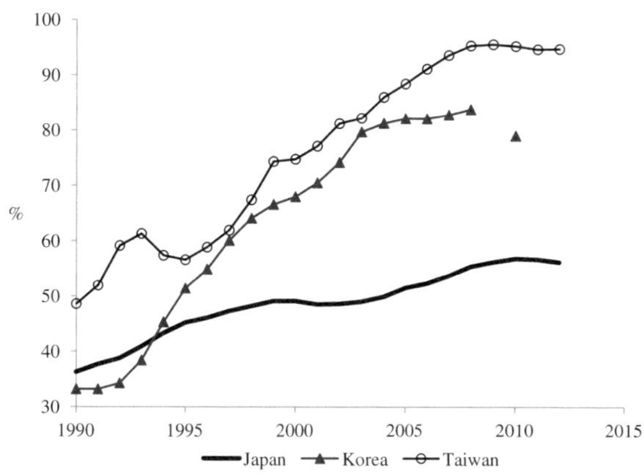

Fig. 5 College enrollment rate of high school graduates. NIPSSR (2013), NSO (2009, 2009), DGBAS

The rate was high for Taiwan, because in that dataset, graduates of vocational high schools were excluded. The rise in college enrollment in Korea in 1990–2005 was especially impressive. Arita (2006) pointed out three characteristics of extraordinary education fever in Korea: its strength is apparent given the higher private education cost that Korean parents pay, relative to other developed countries; it is continuous in the sense that no "cooling down" can be observed; and it is universal in the sense that all social strata are caught in this so-called fever.

Gender differences in college enrollment after 1990 have been small in Eastern Asia. In Japan, the rates of enrollment in 2010 were 57.7 % for males and 56.0 % for females. In Korea and Taiwan, those rate-pairs were 77.6 and 80.5 %, and 94.5 and 96.1 %, respectively.

Table 3 Percentage of private expenditure on education (2009)

Rank	Country	%	Rank	Country	%
1	Chile	41.1	16	Poland	13.3
2	Korea	40.0	17	Spain	12.9
3	Japan	31.9	18	Czech Republic	12.0
4	United Kingdom	31.1	19	Slovenia	11.5
5	United States	28.0	20	France	9.8
6	Australia	26.8	21	Italy	9.3
7	Canada	21.4	22	Iceland	9.2
8	Mexico	21.2	23	Austria	8.6
9	Israel	20.8	24	Portugal	6.5
10	New Zealand	17.4	25	Estonia	5.8
11	Netherlands	16.3	26	Ireland	5.8
12	Slovak Republic	16.1	27	Belgium	5.7
13	Russian Federation	15.2	28	Denmark	4.2
14	Germany	15.0	29	Sweden	2.6
15	Argentina	14.3	30	Finland	2.4

OECD, *Education at a Glance* 2012

Table 3 shows the percentage of educational expenditure paid by private sources. Government support tends to be low in Latin America, Eastern Asia and English-speaking countries. Parents in Korea and Japan pay very high percentages of educational expenditure worldwide, only those in Chile pay a higher percentage. Although data for Taiwan are not available, the situation there should approximate that in Korea and Japan. In this sense, Eastern Asian parents are carrying a greater the financial burden with respect to the cost of children than parents in other developed countries.

2.4.3 Economic Recession and Labor Market Condition

Young people who grew up in periods of rapid economic growth tend to have high aspirations for their future lives. When the economy slows down, however, labor market conditions for young workers become tight. Those who perceive difficulties in achieving their expected standard of living will hesitate to marry and have children (Easterlin 1978; Lutz et al. 2006).

In the case of Japan, the economy has been in a poor condition since the 1990s and the unemployment rate increased sharply from 2 % in 1990 to 5 % in 2003. The tight labor market conditions have seriously discouraged youth in terms of their career achievements. Figure 6 shows the labor force status of college graduates in Japan immediately after graduation. The percentage that had obtained a stable job decreased from 77.8 % in 1988 to 55.0 % in 2003, and then recovered to 71.5 % in 2008. The percentage of those who had obtained a temporary job or who were unemployed increased from 9.4 to 27.1 % between 1988 and 2003. Although the labor market condition for new graduates temporarily improved in 2006–2008, it again worsened due to the 2008 global financial crisis.

Fig. 6 States of college graduates in Japan

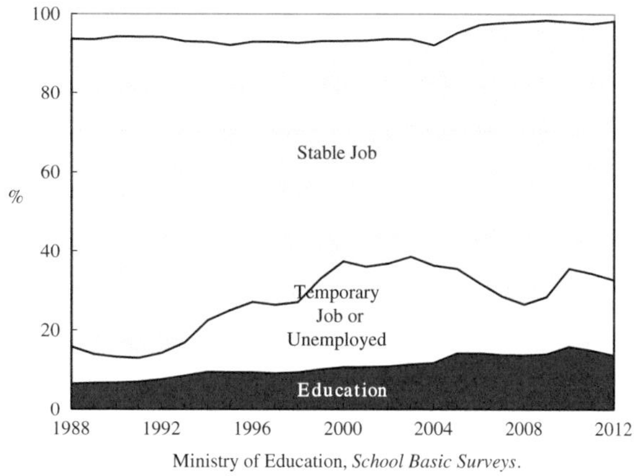

Fig. 7 Expectation on future life of the Japanese

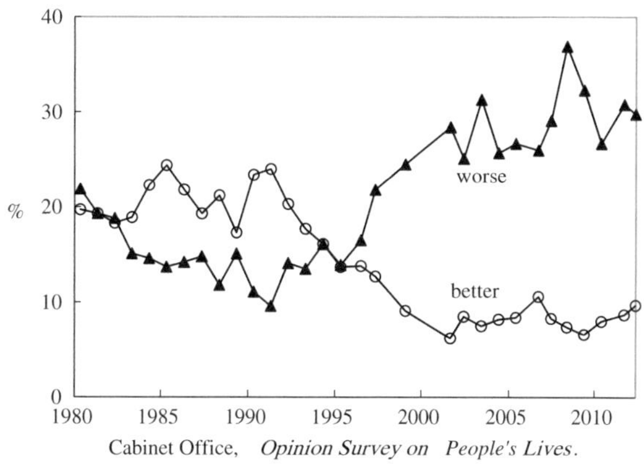

The economic recession is thought to have affected people not only through employment status itself, but also through expected future income. Figure 7 shows the result of an opinion survey conducted by the Cabinet Office of Japan regarding expectations for one's future life. In the late 1980s and early 1990s, more respondents answered "[my life] will get better" than those who answered that it "will get worse." During the 1990s, however, the percentage of respondents who answered "worse" continuously increased, and around 1995 it exceeded the percentage who had answered "better." In June 2012, the pessimistic attitude surpassed the optimistic one by 20 % points. It is thought that such uncertainty about the future is one of the major sources of low fertility in recent Japan.

In Korea, the economic crisis in 1997 brought about a marked change in the labor market. The Kim Dae-Jung government introduced, under the direction of the International Money Fund, a series of neo-liberalist policies meant to secure the "flexibility" of the labor market. While the Korean economy recovered quickly, workers suffered from increases in non-regular employment, job insecurity, and income inequality.

Many Korean social scientists blamed changes following the economic crisis for causing nuptiality and fertility declines. Cha Kyung-Wuk (2005) asserted that a part of the nuptiality decline was due to income decline among women that could not find a job after the crisis. Kim Doo-Sub (2005) asserted that occupational insecurity after the crisis caused fertility decline through the fear of relative deprivation. Eun Ki-Soo (2005) pointed out that fewer job opportunities caused nuptiality decline among males and females alike. Kim Seung-Kwon (2004c) blamed the economic recession and job insecurity for promoting nuptiality and fertility declines.

Unlike Korea, Taiwan did not experience a drastic economic crisis; nonetheless, the Taiwanese may share with the Koreans and Japanese a sense of increased uncertainty and insecurity. The presence and influence of mainland China is especially noteworthy for Taiwan. China's increasing military power, its political conflict with Japan and the United States, and the possibility of economic collapse will have a huge impact on the future of Taiwan.

2.4.4 Female Labor Force Participation

According to Becker (1991), the main cause of family changes since the latter half of the twentieth century has been the increased economic power of women. The increased number of occupational opportunities for women has increased the time they spend on market activities; it has also increased the opportunity cost of children. The declining return from the gender-based division of labor has reduced the benefit of marriage and promoted an increase in the divorce rate. These changes have resulted in an increase in the number of female-headed households, cases of cohabitation, and extramarital births.

The theory predicts the negative impact of female labor force participation on fertility. Actually, a number of empirical studies in Japan have verified at the micro level the negative effect of a wife's work on fertility (Asami et al. 2000; Oyama 2004; Sasai 1998; Shichijo and Nishimoto 2003; Tsuya 1999; Fujino 2002; Yashiro 2000; Yamagami 1999; Yamaguchi 2005). At the macro level, however, the correlation between female labor and fertility among developed countries turned from negative to positive in the 1980s (Billari and Kohler 2002; Atoh 2000).

This paradox can be resolved with a very simple model. Let g be the proportion of working mothers, m be that of all mothers, and w be that of all workers Then, a two-by-two contingency table can be written as follows;

	Not Mother	Mother	
Not Worker	$1 - w - m + g$	$m - g$	$1 - w$
Worker	$w - g$	g	w
	$1 - m$	m	1

For all four cells to be positive, the following condition is necessary in addition to $0 < g < m$ and $0 < g < w$.

$$1 - w - m + g > 0. \tag{6}$$

For the work status of a woman and the presence of a child to negatively correlate, g must be smaller than the expected value of the independence model.

$$g < wm. \tag{7}$$

If we coordinate the proportion of workers (w) on the horizontal axis and with that of mothers (m) on the vertical axis, the area enclosed by a straight line and a hyperbola simultaneously satisfies the two conditions above. Figure 8 shows such areas for $g = 0.2$, 0.4 and 0.6. If we consider g a measure of compatibility, the area moves in the upper-right direction as compatibility improves. Thus, the paradoxical situation can be understood as being a result of increasing compatibility. When women's work and childrearing were less compatible, all of the countries were located at the lower-left region of the graph. However, some countries succeeded in improving compatibility and moved to the upper-right direction. In this way, the positive correlation has appeared at the macro level while the negative correlation is sustained at the micro level.

One implication of Fig. 8 is that the higher the compatibility, the narrower the area in which the micro–macro paradox holds. Then, it is expected that a country with high compatibility may easily escape from the area and the micro-level correlation may become positive. This expectation materialized in Sweden and the United Kingdom, where recent micro-level analyses have shown the positive impact of women's work on fertility (Hoem et al. 2001; Hoorens et al. 2005; Rosenbluth 2007). However, Fig. 8 suggests that in a country with low compatibility—such as Japan and Eastern Asia—there is ample room for fertility decline.

In Japan, improvements of compatibility have not been found to significantly affect fertility. Table 4 shows contingency tables of work status and the presence of a child, among married women aged 30–34. Recently, the age-specific birth rate of this age group has exceeded that of the age 25–29 group to become the age period during which childbearing peaks. The percentage of working mothers (g) increased from 30.2 % in 2004 to 33.8 % in 2007 and to 39.2 % in 2012. This is a result of the increase in labor force participation (w), from 43.1 % in 2004 to 54.6 % in 2012. However, the measure of fertility (m) remained in the narrow range between 76.9 and 78.8 % in those years. While a shift from working non-mothers to working mothers was expected, the percentage of working non-mothers ($w - g$) actually increased in 2004–2007 and remained at around 15 % in 2007–2012.

Figure 9 shows the age patterns of female labor force participation in 2010. The fact that Japan and Korea maintain the so-called M-shaped curve implies that the compatibility between work and family there is relatively low. In Japan, such incompatibility is attributed to persisting attitudes with regard to gender roles, husband's low participation in housework, the characteristics of the labor market,

Fig. 8 Area with negative correlation for different *g*

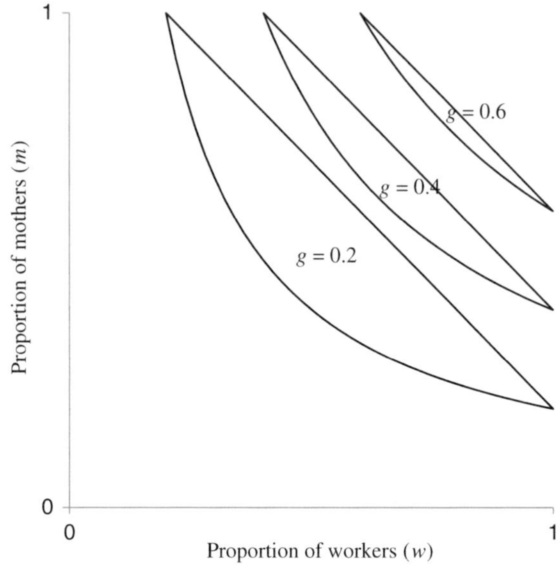

Table 4 Labor force participation and motherhood of married women aged 30–34 (%)

	Not mother	Mother	Total
2004			
Not worker	8.2	48.7	56.9
Worker	12.9	30.2	43.1
Total	21.2	78.8	100
2007			
Not worker	7.5	43	50.5
Worker	15.7	33.8	49.5
Total	23.1	76.9	100
2012			
Not worker	6.5	38.8	45.4
Worker	15.4	39.2	54.6
Total	22	78	100

Ministry of Internal Affairs and Communications, *Employment Status Survey*

and the underdevelopment of family-friendly policy (Atoh and Akachi 2003; Meguro and Nishioka 2000).

While the M-shape was also observed in Taiwan in the 1970s (Sechiyama 1996), the recent pattern shows a monotonous decline for women older than the mid-twenties. This implies that the rapid increase in education attainment among women has had a positive impact on female labor force participation at child-bearing ages. On the other hand, women's education attainment in Japan and Korea has not had the same straightforward impact. In terms of the gender gap in the employment rates of highly educated men and women—as shown in the OECD's report *Employment Outlook 2004*—Korea had the second-largest and

Fig. 9 Labor force participation rates of women in 2010

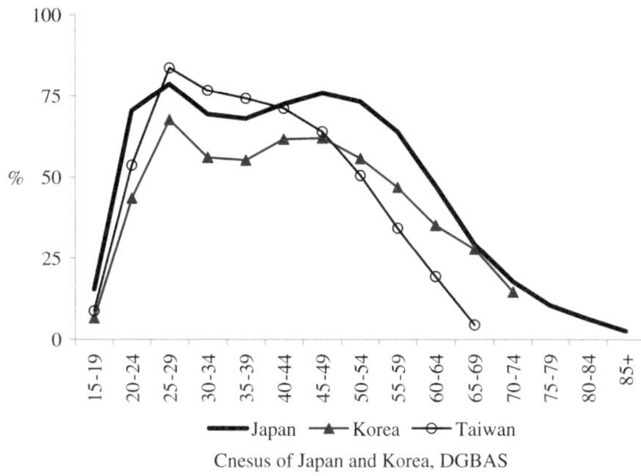

Japan had the third-largest gap, respectively (Choi Eun-Young 2008). Highly educated women in Korea tend to have lower employment rates and a higher probability of retirement at marriage or childbirth than women with low levels of education (Haruki 2006). Sechiyama (1996) attributed the lack of educational effect on women's career attainment to the robustness of patriarchy in Korea.

In addition to the absence of an M-shaped pattern in Taiwan, in the mid-1990s, labor participation among mothers of infants was much higher there than Japan (Shirahase 2007). The fact that the TFR dropped to the lowest level in Taiwan, however, suggests the possibility that an improvement in gender equity and compatibility may not necessarily induce a recuperation of fertility.

2.5 Conclusion

There have been considerable delays both in nuptiality and fertility in Japan. Although the relative importance depends on the choice of time-period, both nuptiality and marital fertility declines have contributed to the decline in TFR. The demand for children in Japan is not as low as in German-speaking countries, as the ideal number of children has never dropped below two. Thus, obstacles to fulfilling the demand for children such as the rising cost of childrearing, increasing uncertainty and job insecurity, female labor force participation and incompatibility between work and family have supposedly brought about low fertility in Japan.

The fertility decline in Korea and Taiwan has been even more marked than in Japan. Compressed modernity (Chang Kyung-Sup 2001, 2002) in these countries seems to have accelerated practically all family changes including fertility decline. However, the response to such socioeconomic changes differs among cultural zones. In addition to the cultural divide between weak and strong family ties, it is useful to discuss yet another cultural divide between Japan and other Eastern Asian countries. The next section focuses on the influence of family patterns and value systems on fertility decline.

3 Low Fertility from a Comparative Perspective

3.1 Introduction

Demographers have been presented with "big pictures" of regional patterns. Hajnal (1965) highlighted the existence of European marriage pattern until the 1940s. Eastern Europe distinguished by the line between Trieste and Leningrad (present-day St. Petersburg) was out of the range of this European pattern. Hajnal (1982) further distinguished Northwest Europe from Southern Europe, Finland, and the Baltic countries, to illuminate the uniqueness of the household formation system in this region. Later achievements in historical demography led Todd to classify family structures in terms of locality and inheritance rules, while additionally considering endogamy/exogamy practice (Todd and Ishizaki 2001). On the cultural divide with respect to fertility, however, the discussion by Reher (1998) on weak family ties in Northwestern Europe and strong family ties in Southwestern Europe seems to be more promising.

Studies on the relationship between value systems and economic development have had a long history, starting with Weber's work on the Protestant ethic. With regard to family systems, Goode (1963) asserted that the Western conjugal family aligned well with the modern industrial system, with its neolocality, limited kin network, emphasis on emotionality between husband and wife, bilateral pattern, equal opportunity among children, loose definition of status obligations, and the economic independence of young couples. He also asserted that the ideology of economic progress and that of egalitarianism are important to the spread of the conjugal family pattern. According to him, the conjugal family pattern has its roots in the individualistic philosophy, and ultimately in Protestantism.

In the 1980s, there was a revival of the classic thesis by Weber with respect to the influence of religious ideology on economic development in Eastern Asia. The impressive economic success of the so-called Four Dragons (i.e., Korea, Taiwan, Hong Kong and Singapore) stimulated studies of Confucian values as the accelerator of development. These studies emphasized the role of education fever and the competitive examination system in addition to the spread of Japanese-style business (Kim Il-Gon 1992; Hayashi 1997).

According to Inglehart and Welzel (2008), modernization goes through two phases. The first phase is industrialization that causes a shift from traditional to secular-rational values. The second stage is the postindustrial phase, which brings about a shift from survival values to self-expression values. While the Confucian value system was very adoptive to industrialization in the 1980s, it does not seem to be adaptive to the recent post-industrialization; the extremely low fertility in Korea and Taiwan is indicative of this. In fact, in the World Value Survey, China, Korea, and Taiwan show lower self-expression value scores than Japan (Inglehart and Norris 2003; Inglehart and Welzel 2008; Halman et al. 2008).

This section examines two cultural divides. The first divide emphasizes the uniqueness of the Northern/Western European family pattern. Because lowest-low fertility has appeared in very different cultural settings (i.e., Southern Europe, Eastern Europe, and Eastern Asia), the phenomenon seems to be a natural response to socioeconomic changes in the post-material era. In this respect, those countries that did not experience lowest-low fertility should be seen as exceptional, and they require explanation. The second divide distinguishes Japan from Confucian countries such as Korea, Taiwan, and China. The recent situation suggests that Japan more closely resembles Europe than Confucian societies in certain respects. The most prominent of which is the feudalism that both Europe and Japan experienced immediately prior to modernization.

3.2 *Cultural Deterministic View of Fertility*

Until the mid-1980s, it was the Scandinavian, Benelux, and German-speaking countries that led fertility decline to the below-replacement level. These countries were characterized by the high prevalence of cohabitation, extramarital births, divorce, single households and female-headed households. The second demographic transition theory (van de Kaa 1987) assumed that the value change from conventional altruistic familism to secularized individualism gave rise to such changes.

In the 1990s, however, the emergence of lowest-low fertility defined as having the TFR of 1.3 or less brought about an upside-down in correlation between fertility and the value system (Kohler et al. 2002). Today, low fertility countries are characterized by low female labor force participation, a robust marriage institution, and strong family ties. Lesthaeghe (2010) asserted that heterogeneity and historical path dependency do not imply the failure of the second demographic transition theory. However, no demographer including the founder of the theory could anticipated such a drastic fertility decline in advance to other symptoms such as cohabitation, extramarital births, divorce and living alone. The connection between low fertility and strong familism created a considerable problem for demographers (Dalla Zuanna 2001; Micheli 2000).

In the early twenty-first century, many countries have escaped lowest-low fertility (Goldstein et al. 2009). Some countries once experienced TFR values lower than 1.3 have regained even the boundary of 1.5 used by McDonald (2005, 2009). However, the cultural divide is still valid. Table 5 shows the TFR values of OECD countries and Taiwan in 2011. It seems that the boundary of 1.6 instead of 1.5 now divides the Group 1 and 2 countries defined by McDonald. The Group 1 countries are English-speaking countries, French and Dutch-speaking Western European countries, and Nordic countries. Luxembourg is the only Group 1 country to have a TFR lower than 1.6. The Group 2 countries comprise Southern/European countries, German-speaking Western European countries, the former Soviet Union countries, and Eastern Asian advanced countries. Here, Cyprus is assumed to be included in Group 2 as a Southern European country. Then, Lithuania is the only exception with a TFR value higher than 1.6. In 2011, four more countries—Slovenia,

Table 5 TFR of OECD Countries and Taiwan (2011)

Country	TFR	Country	TFR
Israel	3.00	Slovenia	1.56
New Zealand	2.06	Switzerland	1.52
Ireland	2.04	Estonia	1.52
Mexico	2.03	Bulgaria	1.51
Turkey	2.02	Luxembourg	1.51
Iceland	2.02	Malta	1.49
France	2.00	Slovak Republic	1.45
United Kingdom	1.97	Austria	1.43
Chile	1.91	Czech Republic	1.43
Sweden	1.90	Italy	1.42
United States	1.89	Greece	1.42
Australia	1.88	Croatia	1.40
Norway	1.88	Japan	1.39
Belgium	1.87	Germany	1.36
Finland	1.83	Portugal	1.36
Lithuania	1.76	Spain	1.36
Netherlands	1.76	Cyprus	1.35
Denmark	1.76	Latvia	1.34
Canada	1.61	Poland	1.30
		Romania	1.25
		Korea	1.24
		Hungary	1.24
		Taiwan	1.07

OECD Family Database, DGBAS

Switzerland, Estonia and Bulgaria—regained the 1.5 level. According to McDonald (2009), the Group 1 countries are characterized by family-friendly institutional arrangements and high gender equity within the family.

The previous section discussed the socioeconomic determinants of fertility decline in Japan and Eastern Asia, such as rising cost of children, growing economic uncertainty and job insecurity, female labor force participation, and the level of work-family balance. Such factors are more or less common among the populations of developed countries. Below-replacement fertility is a natural response to such socioeconomic changes. As a matter of fact, most OECD countries in Table 5 shows TFR values lower than the replacement level. However, the magnitude of response is different between cultures.

3.3 Moderately Low Fertility in Northern/Western Europe

When lowest-low fertility was a phenomenon occurring only in Europe, it was natural to look for features common among the lowest-low fertility countries. However, once lowest-low fertility spread out from Europe, the appropriateness of this attempt became questionable. Since the phenomenon is a natural response to socioeconomic changes in the postindustrial era, those countries that have avoided lowest-low fertility should be seen as exceptional and as requiring explanation. Such countries include the Nordic countries, Western European countries (except for German-speaking countries), and English-speaking countries. Since English-speaking countries are assumed to have the Anglo-Saxon family pattern as the modal model, these countries are referred to as "Northern/Western European countries". From the OECD countries in Table 5, Israel, Mexico, Turkey, and Chile have been excluded. The remaining Southern/Eastern European countries, German-speaking countries, and Eastern Asian countries including Japan are referred as "very low fertility countries".

Reher (1998) asserted that the contrast between weak family ties in Western and Northern Europe and strong family ties in Southern Europe has deep historical roots. In contrast to the Oriental family system, a version of which affected Southern Europe, the Occidental structure is based on the conjugal pair, and women had a higher position in the northern part of the continent. The Reformation changed the meaning of marriage from a sacrament to a civil contract, further enhanced women's position, reduced parental authority, and promoted individualism.

3.3.1 Female Labor Force Participation and Gender Equity

Figure 10 shows the relationship between the female labor force participation rate of 15–49 years in 2008 taken from the ILO Online Database, and the TFR in 2011 taken from the OECD Family Database. For Korea and Taiwan, data from national statistics offices are used. The relationship turned from negative to positive in the mid-1980s (Engelhardt and Prskawetz 2005; Billari and Kohler 2002; Atoh 2000). As mentioned in Sect. 2, this change in aggregate data does not imply an emergent change in the relationship, but rather an increase in unobserved heterogeneity in the compatibility between work and the family. Northern/Western European countries have succeeded in improving that compatibility, and the negative impact of female labor force participation on fertility is thought to have disappeared or even turned positive. In very low fertility countries, however, it is thought that the compatibility remains low and that female labor force participation continues to have the negative impact on fertility.

There are many possible ways to measure gender equity. The United Nations Development Program (UNDP) invented the Gender Inequality Index (GII) in 2010 to replace the old measures such as Gender Development Index (GDI) and Gender Empowerment Measure (GEM). The GII is a synthetic index based on such variables as maternal mortality, adolescent fertility, women's representation in parliament, and gender equity in education and occupation. On the other hand, the Overall Gender Gap (OGG) by the World Economic Forum (WEF) synthesizes various female/male ratios such as labor force participation, income, occupation, education, health, and political participation.

Fig. 10 Female labor participation and fertility

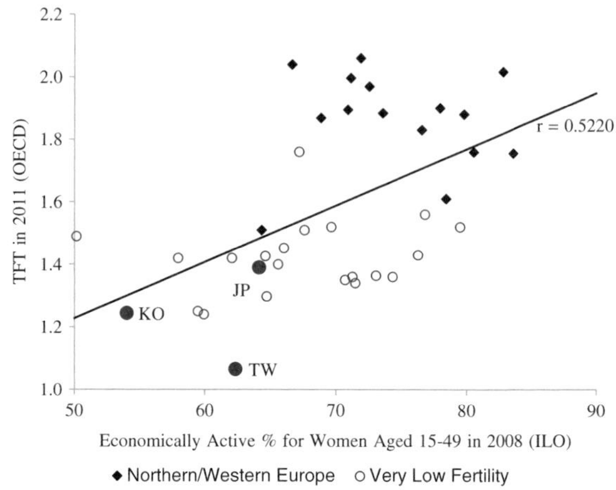

Fig. 11 Gender inequity and fertility (UNDP 2013)

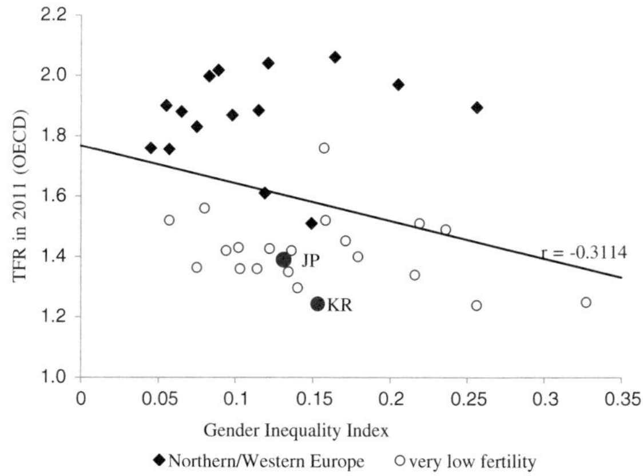

While Fig. 11 shows the correlation between TFR values in Table 5 and GII values according to the UNDP (2013), Fig. 12 shows the correlation with OGG values according to the WEF (2012). Because neither the UNDP nor the WEF presents the value of Taiwan, only 37 countries are plotted in these graphs, compared to 38 countries in Fig. 10. The OGG values more strongly correlate with fertility and more effectively divide Northern/Western Europe and very low fertility countries than the GII can. Note that OGG = 1 implies the perfect equity, and a score lower than 1 implies inequity. Thus, both Figs. 11 and 12 suggest that fertility is low in countries with more serious gender inequity.

Table 6 summarizes the mean of each component used in the GII and the OGG, and their correlation with the TFR. The Eta^2 in this table is the proportion of between-group variance within total variance, and implies the degree of segregation between Group 1 (Northern/Western Europe) and Group 2 (very low fertility countries). Among five components of the GII, secondary education and

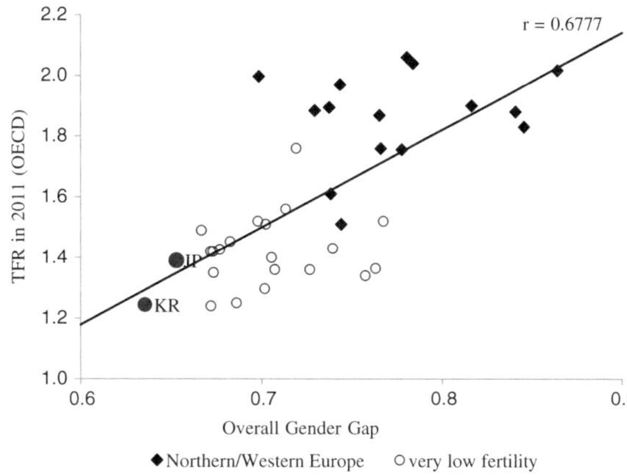

Fig. 12 Gender gap and fertility (WEF 2012)

Table 6 Mean and correlation with TFR of gender equity measures

Components of gender equity	Mean			*Eta*^{2}	Correlation with TFR
	Group 1	Group 2	Total		
Gender inequality index	0.1131	0.1527	0.1366	0.0913	−0.3114
Maternal mortality ratio	9.8667	10.3182	10.1351	0.0010	−0.2163
Adolescent fertility rate	11.8733	12.1091	12.0135	0.0002	0.0732
Seats in national parliament	31.9933	20.4500	25.1297	0.3449	0.5235
Population with at least secondary education	0.9866	0.9420	0.9600	0.1685	0.3990
Labor force participation	0.8325	0.7565	0.7873	0.2586	0.5146
Overall gender gap	0.7753	0.6995	0.7302	0.4691	0.6777
Labor force participation	0.8733	0.8009	0.8303	0.1792	0.4180
Wage equality for similar work	0.6927	0.5841	0.6281	0.3799	0.5837
Estimated earned income	0.8227	0.6241	0.7046	0.4817	0.5456
Legislators, senior officials and managers	0.5157	0.4355	0.4667	0.0790	0.3613
Professional and technical workers	1.1121	1.2232	1.1800	0.0474	−0.0410
Literacy rate	1.0000	0.9955	0.9973	0.0589	0.2873
Enrolment in primary education	1.0027	1.0000	1.0011	0.0230	0.0266
Enrolment in secondary education	1.0100	1.0086	1.0092	0.0006	0.0075
Enrolment in tertiary education	1.3687	1.2736	1.3122	0.0348	0.3516
Sex ratio at birth	0.9473	0.9409	0.9435	0.1641	0.4923
Healthy life expectancy	1.0460	1.0791	1.0657	0.2156	−0.3606
Women in parliment	0.4780	0.2791	0.3597	0.2568	0.4472
Women in ministerial positions	0.5640	0.2791	0.3946	0.2235	0.4081
Years with female head of state	0.1727	0.0364	0.0916	0.1599	0.5408

Group 1 Australia, Belgium, Canada, Denmark, Finland, France, Iceland, Ireland, Luxembourg, Netherlands, New Zealand, Norway, Sweden, U.K., U.S

Group 2 Austria, Bulgaria, Croatia, Cyprus, Czech, Estonia, Germany, Greece, Hungary, Italy, Japan, Korea, Latvia, Lithuania, Malta, Poland, Portugal, Romania, Slovakia, Slovenia, Spain, Switzerland

Source OECD Family Database, Human Development Report 2013, Gender Gap Report 2012

labor force participation are female/male ratios. All the components of the OGG are female/male ratios.

Actually, the strongest correlation with fertility can be found in the synthetic measure of the OGG. The correlation with fertility tends to be strong for economic equality and weak for educational and health equality. Some measures of political equality—such as seats in parliament in the GII and years with a female head in the OGG—also show a strong correlation with fertility. The largest divergence between Groups 1 and 2 can be found in the female/male ratio of income, followed by the OGG. Again, segregation is weak in educational and health equality. Thus, it is primarily economic gender equality that supports moderately low fertility in Northern/Western Europe and the uniqueness of these countries. Political gender equality has secondary importance, followed by equality in education and health (Table 6).

3.3.2 Premarital Home-Leaving

Another prominent feature of Northern/Western Europe and their descendants is relatively early age at which children leave home. In these countries in the pre-industrial era, young men and women left the parental home before marriage to work as servants (Reher 1998; Wall 1989). The tradition of the majority of men and women leaving home before marriage remains today (Billari et al. 2001). Premarital home-leaving is thought to promote union formation through both consensual union and formal marriage, while Southern European adolescents suffer from "postponement syndrome," which discourages autonomy and weakens their ability to make decisions in their own lives (Dalla Zuanna 2001; Livi-Bacci 2001). As shown in Fig. 13, Japan occupies a unique position that men leave as early as their Northern European counterparts, while women leave as late as their Southern European counterparts. However, since late home-leaving among individuals of either sex discourages union formation, Japan may suffer from the same problem as Southern Europe.

Although median ages at home-leaving in Korea and Taiwan are not available, these two countries are expected to have the same pattern as Japan (Suzuki 2011). Because of military conscription, Korean and Taiwanese men are supposed to leave their parental homes earlier than women. As seen in Sect. 2, the percentage of single women in their late twenties in Korea and Taiwan has exceeded that in Japan. The percentage of women aged 25–29 living alone, according to the 2010 census, was 17.1 % in Japan and 15.6 % in Korea. Although data pertaining to the percentage of young women living alone by age cannot be found in the Taiwanese census, Yang Ching-Li et al. (2012) estimated the percentage to be as low as 2.08 % in 2003–2005. Thus, it is likely in Korea and Taiwan that single women stay longer at the parental household and leave later than do Japanese women.

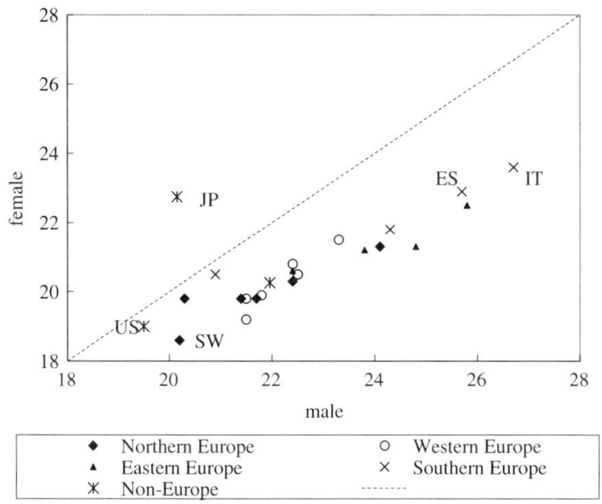

Fig. 13 Median age at home-leaving of cohorts born around 1960. Billari et al. (2001), Goldscheider et al. (1994), Ravanera et al. (1995), Suzuki (2003)

Fig. 14 Extramarital birth and fertility in 2009

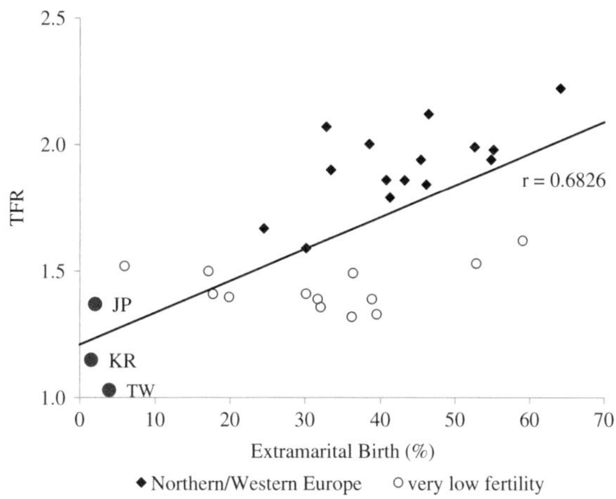

3.3.3 Extramarital Births

Figure 14 shows the relation in 2009 between the percentage of extramarital births and fertility; these data were taken from the OECD Family Database and the Directorate General of Budget, Accounting, and Statistic (DGBAS) of Taiwan. The increase in cohabitation and extramarital births during the second demographic transition could be attributed to weak familism in Northern/Western Europe. It is possible that the notion of marriage as a civil contract rather than a sacrament and the emphasis on individual autonomy helped disconnect reproduction from marriage. While the figure suggests that the increase in extramarital births does not necessarily lead to fertility recovery, a percentage of 20 % or more seems to be a condition essential to moderately low fertility. In fact, the recent fertility recovery in Southern European countries is accompanied by the delayed second demographic transition—namely, the spread of cohabitation, extramarital births, and marital instability (Billari 2008). Other elements of the second demographic transition, meanwhile, have already taken place in Eastern Asian advanced countries; only the increase in extramarital births cannot be observed in this region (Lesthaeghe 2010).

3.3.4 Enrollment in Childcare

Figure 15 shows the correlation between early childhood services for those under age three, and the TFR in 2010 as per the OECD Family Database. Data for Taiwan were not available. Unlike in low fertility countries where childcare is the mother's supreme role, Northern/Western European countries developed non-parental childcare activities involving baby-sitters, tutors, childcare workers and other professionals. It is thought that weak parent–child ties within this region have had an important role in promoting the use of early childhood services and thus improved the compatibility between work and the family. In contrast, countries with strong family ties are still clinging to maternal care.

Although Japan and Korea show higher daycare enrollment (28.3 and 37.7 %, respectively) than other very low fertility countries, these rates are still lower than those of most Northern/Western European countries. According to the Third National Family Survey in 2003 by NIPSSR, 82.9 % of Japanese wives agreed with "A mother should not work, but should take care of her child for 3 years after birth." Such an emphasis on the mother's supreme role could be the factor that curbs the effect that childcare service would otherwise have on fertility. According to Retherford and Ogawa (2006), Japan's low enrollment rate of young children in daycare centers owes not to a short supply of service but to mothers' desire to raise their children on their own. The low daycare enrollment rate in Korea, together with the M-shaped pattern, suggests that mother–child ties in Korea are as strong as those in Japan.

As has been seen thus far, countries with a Northern/Western European cultural background are characterized by weak family ties, high compatibility between work and the family, the relatively high position of women, early independence among children, weakened marriage institution, and the participation of nonfamily members in childbearing. Because of these distinctive family patterns, those countries could avoid lowest-low fertility even with postmodern economic and social changes. Gender equity was achieved swiftly in those countries, in both the formal and informal spheres, because women's position in antiquity was already high. Union formation was not overly delayed in terms of prolonged human investment, given the norms of early home-leaving and economic independence. The decline in marriage was immediately compensated by an increase in cohabitation and extramarital births. The compatibility between work and the family quickly improved, because non-maternal childcare activities were common.

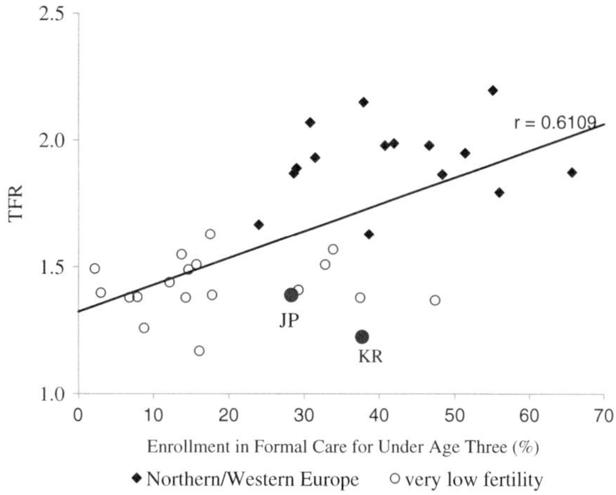

Fig. 15 Childcare enrollment and fertility in 2010

3.4 Extremely Low Fertility in Confucian Countries

Table 7 summarizes the lowest TFR value experienced by advanced countries. Some countries such as the Czech Republic, the Slovak Republic, Italy, and Spain have experienced TFR values lower than 1.2. However, neither Japan nor any European country has experienced TFR values lower than 1.1. On the other hand, Korea recorded a TFR of 1.08 in 2005, and Taiwan 0.895 in 2010. Thus, there seems to be another cultural divide, with Korea and Taiwan on one side and the other OECD countries on the other. While Korean and Taiwanese families are offspring of a Confucian family, other countries can be seen as offspring of a feudal family. Feudalism is a loose integration of feudal lords that had their own military powers and laws and existed only in Europe and Japan immediately before modernization. In this sense, Japan was not a Confucian society but a feudal one just like European countries.

Although feudalism existed also in ancient China, the political system there shifted to a centralized agricultural bureaucracy (Cumings 2005) after the Qin dynasty. The elaborated imperial examination system in the Tang dynasty marked the establishment of the familistic Confucian social system in China. The Yi dynasty of Korea enforced Confucianism among the Korean people, and by the 19th century, Korean society had become more Confucian than China itself.

These countries sharply contrasted with Japan in the early nineteenth century. The decentralized and loosely integrated political system of Japan allowed for competition between feudal lords (daimyos). Since the master-servant relationship was the principle underpinning society, loyalty was more highly valued than filial piety, which was the most fundamental Confucian value. Since an imperial examination system had not been introduced to Japan, society there was more closed in terms of social mobility. On the other hand, a Japanese family household (i.e.) could include a member who was not related by blood. This feudal and less familistic value system prevented nepotism and promoted the rule of law.

Table 7 Recorded lowest TFR in OECD countries and Taiwan

Country	TFR	Year	Country	TFR	Year
Iceland	1.93	2002	Austria	1.33	2001
New Zealand	1.89	2002	Portugal	1.32	2007
Ireland	1.85	1995	Estonia	1.28	1998
United States	1.74	1976	Japan	1.26	2005
Australia	1.73	2001	Germany	1.24	1994
France	1.66	1994	Greece	1.24	1999
Norway	1.66	1984	Hungary	1.24	2011
United Kingdom	1.63	2001	Poland	1.22	2003
Belgium	1.51	1985	Slovenia	1.20	2003
Finland	1.50	1973	Italy	1.19	1995
Sweden	1.50	1999	Slovak Republic	1.19	2002
Canada	1.49	2000	Spain	1.16	1998
Netherlands	1.47	1983	Czech Republic	1.13	1999
Denmark	1.38	1983	Korea	1.08	2005
Luxembourg	1.38	1985	Taiwan	0.90	2010
Switzerland	1.38	2001			

OECD Family Database, DGBAS

The sharp contrast between Japan and other Eastern Asian societies led to a view that Japan stands as an isolated civilization, while Korea and Vietnam are included in Chinese (Confucian) civilization (Huntington 1996). According to Eisenstadt (1996), Japan is the only non-axial civilization that has not been alienated or absorbed into one of the axial civilizations. Nakane (1967) also stated that Japanese society is very different from that of China, India, or Europe in emphasizing social groups based on location. On the other hand, many scholars including E. H. Norman, T. Persons, and E. Durkheim pointed out similarities in social structure and historical development between Japan and Europe (Eisenstadt 1996). In Japan, Umezao (1957) asserted that Japan and Europe are special places where "autogenic succession" proceeded to prepare the bourgeoisie and capitalism.

In the feudal family system, the parent–child relationship and conjugal relations were seen from rights and obligations between autonomous persons. Although family relations were by no means egalitarian, inferiors like children or the wife were thought to have their own rights in addition to obligations. The position of women was relatively high, and the idea of contracts was common in family relations. If Northern/Western Europe was the most typical case of a feudal family system, then Southern Europe and Japan can be seen as cases of a feudal family influenced by patriarchal and authoritarian patterns of the Roman family, Islamic family or Confucian family.

The Confucian family pattern contrasts with feudal family patterns. In the former, filial piety is an absolute obligation, as it is considered a law of nature. Within the pattern, a child was totally powerless before the father, and the idea of a contract was out of the question. This was very different from the Samurai family pattern in Japan, in which filial piety was seen as the returning of a debt to the

Table 8 Family pattern immediately before modernization

	China	Korea	Japan
Ideology	Filial piety	Filial piety	Loyalty
Trust on non-family	Low	Low	High
Woman's position	Rigid segregation	Rigid segregation	Relatively equal
Kinship group	Patrilineal	Patrilineal	Bilateral or weakly patrilineal
Marriage	Exogamy	Exogamy	Endogamy
Adoption	Within clan, generation is considered	Within clan, generation is considered	Free
Inheritance	Equal among sons	Weak primogeniture	Primogeniture
Household structure	Joint family or circulation of parent	Stem family	Stem family

parents (Kawashima 1957). While the family was the basic model for all social organization in Confucian society, the essence of the Samurai family stemmed from a master–servant relation (Goode 1963).

Fukuyama (1995) attributed the difference between the high-trust Japanese society and low-trust Chinese society to the relative strength of familism. The Chinese people tend not to trust nonfamily members, and this makes it difficult to establish a huge enterprise in Chinese societies. Traditional communities in China lacked solidity to cooperate for a large project. In Japan, familism was weaker, and so nepotism was more carefully avoided. Loyalty to nonfamily groups such as community and the feudal government was emphasized, which in turn fostered patriotism and nationalism.

The contrast between the Japanese feudal family and the Confucian family is made evident when one examines the position of women immediately prior to modernization. Westerners visiting Japan in the eighteenth and nineteenth centuries found that the position of Japanese women was higher than that in other Asian societies, especially in China (Screech 2005; Murphey 2009; Perry 1856; Griffis 1876).

Table 8 summarizes the family patterns in China, Korea, and Japan in the nineteenth century. As mentioned, filial piety was the fundamental ideology of a Confucian society. Although trust in others tends to be low within Confucian society, Korea is an exceptional case, in that it has successfully developed very large enterprises. Women in Confucian society were rigidly segregated from the formal productive sector. In Confucian society, both men and women succeed father's surname, and it does not change even after marriage. Nakane (1970) emphasized the difference between "*dozoku*" in Japan and the Chinese patrilineal clan. In Japan, an adopted son or a married daughter lost his or her membership to the family of orientation. Although more emphasis is placed on the paternal line, both paternal and maternal lines are considered integral to kinship.

While marriage within the paternal clan was strictly prohibited in Confucian societies, adoptions were always executed within the clan. On the other hand, the

Japanese family was more interested in sustaining the family name and property rather than the blood line. Thus, even an unrelated man could be adopted as the designated heir. Although there are some similarities between Japan and Korea in terms of inheritance norms and household structure, the contrast between Japan and Confucian societies is more impressive.

3.5 Gender Equity in Eastern Asia

While it is plausible that the position of women in the nineteenth century was higher in Japan than in Korea or China, the present-day situation is more difficult to evaluate. As shown in Table 9, Japan has higher equality than Korea or China in terms of the UNDP's GII. On the other hand, the WEF's OGG suggests that China has higher equality than Japan or Korea. The difference comes from the components and weights inherent in these synthetic indices. China's higher inequality in the GII is due to greater maternal mortality, higher adolescent fertility, and a lower percentage of women finished secondary education. Although China's literacy, education, birth, and health scores are low, the overall OGG score is high because it contains more components pertaining to economic and political equality. As mentioned, economic and political equality are more closely related to fertility than educational and health equality. It is possible that the current situation in China can prevent fertility there from declining to the extremely low levels as seen in Korea and Taiwan (Table 9).

According to McDonald (2000), however, it is the combination of low gender equity within the family and high gender equity outside the family that creates very low fertility. If a strong preference for sons (shown in Fig. 16) reflects low gender equity within the family, then China's TFR could drop to extremely low levels. The figure clearly shows the difference between Japan and Confucian countries. While Korea's sex ratio at birth was recently normalized, Taiwan's convergence is slow in coming. This suggests that traditional Confucian values are more robust in Taiwan than in Korea.

Although the UNDP does not calculate indices for Taiwan, DGBAS (2013) asserts that the GII of Taiwan in 2012 was 0.053, making it the second-lowest score, surpassed only by the Netherlands (0.045). Considering Taiwan's high compatibility between work and family as mentioned in Sect. 2, it is plausible that Taiwan's gender equity in the formal sector is higher than that of Japan or Korea. However, the results of opinion surveys suggest that the Taiwanese people have a more traditional attitude toward family relationships than do the Japanese, Koreans, and mainland Chinese. Table 10 compares the results of East Asian Social Survey modules included in the JGSS, KGSS, and CGSS (i.e., the General Social Surveys in Japan, Korea, and China) and the TSCS (Taiwan Social Change Survey) in 2006. In seven of 10 questions, the Taiwanese respondents showed the

Table 9 Gender equity in Japan, Korea and China

	Japan	Korea	China	order
Gender Inequality Index	0.13	0.15	0.21	J < K < C
Maternal mortality ratio	5.0	16.0	37.0	J < K < C
Adolescent fertility rate	6.0	5.8	9.1	K < J < C
Seats in national parliament	13.4	15.7	21.3	J < K < C
Population with at least secondary education	0.97	0.87	0.78	C < K < J
Labor force participation	0.69	0.69	0.85	C < J < K
Overall Gender Gap	0.65	0.64	0.69	K < J < C
Labor force participation	0.73	0.73	0.88	J = K < C
Wage equality for similar work	0.60	0.54	0.66	K < J < C
Estimated earned income	0.55	0.44	0.65	K < J < C
Legislators, senior officials and managers	0.10	0.11	0.20	J < K < C
Professional and technical workers	0.87	0.69	1.08	K < J < C
Literacy rate	1.00	1.00	0.94	C < J = K
Enrolment in primary education	1.00	0.99	1.00	K < J = C
Enrolment in secondary education	1.00	0.99	0.97	C < K < J
Enrolment in tertiary education	0.89	0.72	1.10	K < J < C
Sex ratio at birth	0.94	0.93	0.88	C < K < J
Healthy life expectancy	1.07	1.09	1.05	C < J < K
Women in parliament	0.12	0.19	0.27	J < K < C
Women in ministerial positions	0.13	0.14	0.13	J = C < K
Years with female head of state	0.00	0.02	0.08	J < K < C

Source Human Development Report 2013, Gender Gap Report 2012

Fig. 16 Sex ratio at birth

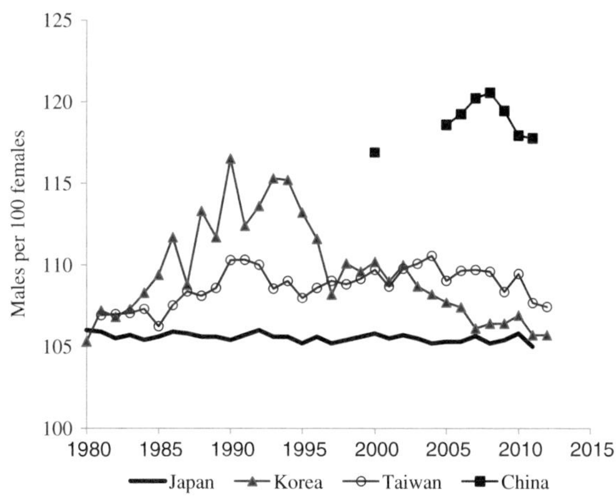

strongest familism. Thus, there could be a huge gap in gender relations between the formal sector and the family sector, and this may be causing extremely low fertility.

Table 10 Familism in Eastern Asia

Percent of "strongly agree"	Taiwan	Korea	Japan	China
One should give priority to the happiness and benefit of the family than one's own	28.5	21.5	4.4	9.3
A child should pay effort to make parents to be proud of	34.2	18.3	2.7	19.5
A wife should help her husband's family when both families need help	8.2	7.8	1.5	3.2
Three generation household is desirable	72.2	58.4	67.5	59.5
The eldest son should inherit more property	3.0	6.1	1.5	2.8
A child who took care of parents should inherit more property	8.8	26.1	9.4	9.6
A father's authority should be respected whatever the situation is	25.9	31.1	3.9	17.6
It is more important for a wife to support her husband's work than her own work	12.8	12.8	1.8	5.1
A husband should work outside and a wife should keep the house	15.4	9.7	2.2	5.6
It is allowed to lay off women before men in a recession	2.0	1.8	1.0	1.5

Source Iwai and Yasuda (2009)

3.6 Conclusion

It seems that below-replacement fertility is a natural response to such postindustrial socioeconomic changes as slow economic growth, tight labor market conditions for young workers, high job insecurity, and increased female labor force participation. The degree of fertility decline may depend on both the magnitude of socioeconomic changes and the vulnerability of families within each society. It is likely that socioeconomic changes were most drastic in the Eastern European and former Soviet Union countries as they experienced the transition to a market economy. According to UNPD (2013), the life expectancy in Russia dropped from 69.15 in 1985–1990 to 64.97 in 2000–2005. However, Russia's lowest ever TFR was 1.16 recorded in 1999 (Goldstein et al. 2009). Thus, the extremely low TFR values such as 1.08 in Korea and 0.895 in Taiwan seem to be a result from the vulnerability of the Confucian family pattern to postindustrial socioeconomic changes.

In addition to the emergence of fertility decline which no demographic theory had correctly anticipated, Eastern Asian countries have difficulties to cope with low fertility, due to the fear for overpopulation, conservatism that supports the male breadwinner model, and the small budgets of neo-liberalist governments. While Japan established pro-natal policy in the 1990s and Korea and Taiwan started to do so in the 2000s, China sustains anti-natal policy in spite of a below-replacement fertility rate. Section 4 discusses those political developments in four Eastern Asian countries.

4 Politics of Low Fertility in Japan and Eastern Asia

4.1 Introduction

In the course of industrialization, the family lost its position as the unit of economic production. Since then, various functions that were once assigned solely to the family have been shared by the public and market sectors. Because childrearing is considered one of the most basic functions of the family, governments have tended to be slower to intervene in that area than in economic support to and care for the elderly, or in labor force participation by married women.

It is assumed that Japan belongs to the "liberal regime" of welfare states, along with English-speaking developed countries (Gauthier 2002). This type, according to the scheme of Espen-Andersen, is characterized by a low level of family support and reliance on the market to provide childcare services. Korea and Taiwan also supposedly have liberal regimes, given the neo-liberalistic attitude of their respective governments. However, TFR values of Japan, Korea, and Taiwan are much lower than those of English-speaking developed countries. It is apparent that these countries, especially the United States, cannot serve as role models in terms of family policy. Instead, Japan, Korea, and Taiwan have been attempting to introduce policy measures in Northern/Western welfare states in spite of their neoliberalism.

4.2 Fertility Policy of Japan

4.2.1 Overview of Political Development

Japan experienced its first demographic transition in the 1950s and arrived at a below-replacement fertility level in 1956 with a TFR of 2.22 and an NRR (Net Reproduction Rate) of 0.99. However, the TFR fluctuated around the replacement level until 1973 when a TFR of 2.14 and an NRR of 1.01 were recorded. The time between the late 1950s and the early 1970s comprised the "golden age of the family", with rapid economic growth, parental altruism, and successful gender role divisions between male breadwinners and fulltime housewives.

Japan's second demographic transition started in the mid-1970s; its TFR crossed the boundary of 1.8 in 1978. However, Japanese demographers assumed, as did those of in other developed countries, that below-replacement fertility was a temporary phenomenon caused by the delay in childbearing, and that the TFR would be restored to replacement levels within several decades. As shown in Fig. 17, medium fertility variants of official population projections conducted in the 1980s assumed that TFR values would eventually converge to 2.0 or higher. The turning point was in 1989, when Japan's TFR hit its historically low level of 1.57. Japanese demographers once believed that the TFR of 1.58 in 1966 prompted

Fig. 17 Observed and projected total fertility rate in Japan

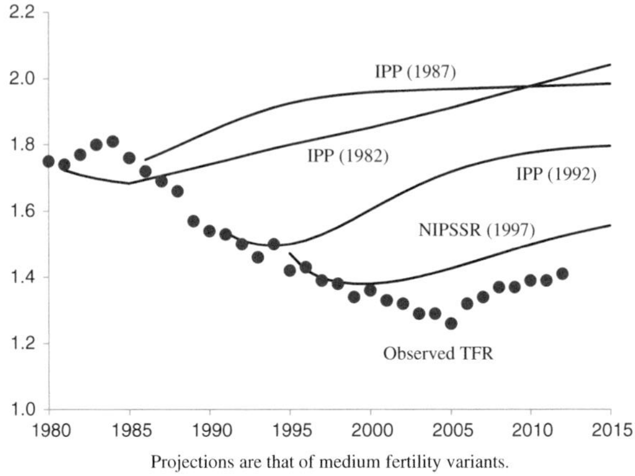

by *hinoeuma* superstition (suggesting a girl born in this year would be evil) was so abnormal that the TFR would never drop below this level. After this "1.57 shock", official population projections ceased to assume replacement levels in the predictable future.

Table 11 summarizes the development of pro-natal policy measures in Japan. It was difficult for political leaders to introduce pro-natal measures, given bad memories from the military era (Atoh 2000). However, the 1.57 shock was enough to convince political leaders of the necessity of pro-natal policy. The government launched in 1990 an inter-ministry committee to assemble measures to cope with declining fertility. In 1991, the amount of child allowance was raised, while the period of payment was shortened to maintain budgets. The Childcare Leave Law was established in May 1991 and enforced in April 1992.

In December 1994, the government publicized the Angel Plan for the 1994–1999 period. The program emphasized the compatibility between work and childcare, and public support for childrearing. As a part of this program, amendments to the Childcare Leave Law were made in 1994 to support income and exempt social security premium payment. In 1997, a major reformation was made to the Child Welfare Law to provide working mothers with satisfactory daycare services.

In December 1999, the government released the New Angel Plan for the 1999–2004 period. This document asserted the need to improve gender equity and working conditions. In May 2000, an amendment to the Childcare Leave Law determined that 40 % of wages should be paid during the leave. The child allowance, previously available only for children under 3 years of age, was expanded to cover preschoolers as well. In July 2001, the cabinet adopted the "Zero Waiting List for Daycare Program" as a political goal.

The Next Generation Law, enacted in July 2003, required local governments and large companies to create their own programs to foster new generations. At the same time, the Law for Measures to Cope with Decreasing Children Society ordered the Cabinet Office to prepare new measures to prevent further rapid

Table 11 Pro-natal policy interventions in Japan

Year	Policy measures
1991	Government's guideline "Toward Satisfactory Conditions for Healthy Childbearing"
	Amendments to Child Allowance Law
	Childcare Leave Law
1994	Angel Plan (1994–1999)
	Amendments to Childcare Leave Law
1997	Amendments to Child Welfare Law
1999	New Angel Plan (2000–2004)
2000	Amendments to Childcare Leave Law
	Amendments to Child Allowance Law
2002	Ministry of Health "Measures for Decreasing Children Plus One"
2003	Law for measures to support the development of the next generation
	Law for measures to cope with decreasing children society
	Amendment to Child Allowance Law
2004	Support plan for parents and children (2005–2009)
2006	New policy to cope with low fertility
2007	Important strategy to support children and the family
2010	Visions for children and childrearing (2010–2014)
2012	Three new laws for childcare

decline in fertility. An expansion of the child allowance, to cover children in the third grade of primary school, was enforced in April 2004.

In December 2004, the government announced the Support Plan for Parents and Children (New–New Angel Plan) for the 2004–2009 period. The document emphasized the role of local governments and companies in providing childcare supports and improving gender equity. In addition, that document pointed out the importance of economic independence among youth. From fiscal year 2006, the child allowance was again expanded, to cover children in the sixth grade. In addition, the Support Plan for Mothers' Reentry to the Labor Market was implemented. That plan included such measures as starting a course at vocational schools for mothers who are reentering the work force, helping mothers who are attempting to start businesses, and running "Mothers' Hello Works" for job-seeking mothers.

In June 2006, the government announced the New Policy to Cope with Low Fertility. The monthly cash benefit of the child allowance was raised from JPY 5,000 to JPY 10,000 until the third birthday of the child. The Important Strategy to Support Children and the Family, announced in 2007, focused on the issue of compatibility between work and the family. The agreed-upon Work-Life Balance Charter proposed to raise the employment rate and productivity while reducing the number of temporary workers, to shorten working hours while seeking better family life, and to improve flexibility and gender equity in the workplace.

These measures were mainly introduced by the coalition government comprising the Liberal Democratic Party (LDP) and the New Komei Party (NKP), which took power between 1999 and 2009. In 2009, however, the Democratic Party of Japan (DPJ) won the election and formed a coalition with People's New Party and the Social Democratic Party, although the latter withdrew in May 2010.

In January 2010, the government publicized a new action program called Visions for Children and Childrearing. It included certain election promises of the DPJ such as expansion of the child allowance program. The party promised to increase the monthly benefit from JPY 10,000 to JPY 26,000 and to abandon the means test. It turned out, however, that such an increase would be impossible, owing to budget constraints. The document also proposed to integrate daycare center and kindergarten to improve childcare services. Three new laws for childcare passed in August 2012 transferred the authority of permission and supervision of childcare service from the Ministry of Health (daycare centers) and Ministry of Education (kindergarten) to the Cabinet Office and prefectural governments.

4.2.2 Child Allowance

In Japan, the child allowance started in 1971. At that time, eligibility was limited only to children of the third and higher birth order, less than 5 years old, and whose parents did not exceed the income threshold. The birth order limit was loosened to the second child (1985) and to the first child (1990). The age limit was increased in 1974 to all preschoolers, but lowered again to 3 years in 1985. The age limit was increased in 2000 to the entrance to primary school, in 2004 to the third grade, in 2006 to graduation of primary school, and in 2010 to graduation from junior high school.

In the fiscal years of 1992–2006, the monetary amounts were JPY 10,000 or YPY 5,000 per month, according to birth order. A means test was used while the LDP and NKP were in power. Approximately 85 % of children received the allowance before the means test was temporarily abolished in 2010 (Suzuki 2006; Boling 2007; Tanaka 2008).

As mentioned, the DPJ had an ambitious plan to increase the monthly benefit to JPY 26,000 and abandon the means test. However, the new act passed in March 2010 stated that only JPY 13,000 would be paid, owing to budget constraints, although the age limit was increased and the means test was indeed abandoned (Table 12). The DPJ eventually abandoned the election promise and decided in 2011 to return to the previous formula. This political failure has supposedly damaged the Japanese people's trust in governmental support to childrearing.

While the wife's income may have a negative impact on fertility due to the opportunity cost, the income of other household members will increase fertility through the income effect. Thus, the child allowance can be considered the additional income of the husband or household. Then, the effect of the child allowance can be evaluated by examining the coefficient of income in a fertility

Table 12 Child allowance in Japan since 2007

Age	Birth order	2007.4–2010.3	2010.4–2011.9	2011.10–2012.3	2012.4–
0–2	All	10,000 yen	13,000 yen	15,000 yen	15,000 yen
3–12	1st and 2nd	5,000 yen	13,000 yen	10,000 yen	10,000 yen
3–12	3rd+	10,000 yen	13,000 yen	15,000 yen	15,000 yen
13–15	All	0 yen	13,000 yen	10,000 yen	10,000 yen
Means text		Yes	No	No	Yes

Table 13 Estimated effects of child allowance in Japan (10,000 yen)

Literature	Yamagami (1999)	Oi (2004)	Morita (2006)	Hoshi (2007)
Income	Husband's annual income	Husband's monthly income	Logarithmic husband's monthly income	Logarithmic household annual income
Coefficient	0.00244	0.01	0.043	0.372
Increase in TFR	0.02928	0.01	0.00193	0.01902

function. Table 13 summarizes such coefficients and the increase in TFR prompted by an additional JPY 10,000 to the monthly income (Table 13).

Yamagami (1999) conducted a multiple regression analysis on the number of children and found that a JPY 10,000 increase in the husband's annual income would raise the number of children by 0.00244. Then, the addition of JPY 120,000 would increase fertility by $12 \times 0.00244 = 0.02928$. An OLS estimate of Oi (2004) suggests that an additional JPY 10,000 in husband's monthly income would increase the number of children by 0.01. The results of Morita (2006) were less encouraging: the elasticity of the number of children to the husband's monthly income was 0.043. Since the average income was JPY 432 thousand, an additional JPY 10,000 implies an increase of $10/432 = 2.313\ \%$. This change in the husband's income results in a very small increase in fertility, by $0.02313 \times 0.043 = 0.09946\ \%$. Because the average number of children was 1.955, this means that the number of children would increase by a mere $1.955 \times 0.00099646 = 0.00193$ persons. Finally, Hoshi (2007) found that the coefficient of the logarithmic household annual income to the number of children was 0.372. Because the average income was JPY 6,249 thousand, an additional JPY 120,000 would prompt a $120/6249 = 1.92\ \%$ increase in children. This means that, the number of children would increase by $0.372 \times \ln(1.0192) = 0.01902$. On the whole, the income effect on fertility is so small that it would be difficult to increase the TFR significantly through the provision of a child allowance. However, the policy has symbolic meaning in addition to real benefits (McDonald 2008). The provision of a child allowance is an important message that the government wants to help parents in raising their children.

4.2.3 Maternity Leave and Childcare Leave

Under Japan's current Labor Standard Law, a female worker can take 14 weeks leave, 6 weeks before and 8 weeks after childbirth. She receives JPY 420,000 from the health insurance system, which is meant to cover hospital costs. In addition to this one-time cash benefit, the health insurance can cover two-thirds of the woman's wage during the maternity leave, if her employer does not pay any wage. According to the National Fertility Survey in 2010, 21.4 % of all mothers used maternity leave at their first birth. That percentage was 87.1 % for mothers who remained as permanent workers (NIPSSR 2012b).

In Japan, childcare leave was established in 1991. Under the current system, either a mother or a father can take childcare leave until the first birthday of the child. A parent who experiences difficulty in using daycare services can prolong the leave for an additional 6 months. A parent during childcare leave receives the benefit equivalent to 30 % of the wage. She or he also receives 20 % of the wage upon reinstatement to work. According to the National Fertility Survey in 2010, 16.7 % of all mothers and 75.5 % of permanently working mothers took childcare leave after the first birth (NIPSSR 2012b).

Several studies evaluated the effect of childcare leave on fertility in Japan. Table 14 shows the partial regression coefficients in four studies. Since each coefficient b is supposed to show a log-odds ratio of fertility between a female who can take childcare leave and one who cannot, $\exp(b)$ provides an odds ratio. Because Shigeno and Matsuura (2003) and Yamaguchi (2005) each analyzed fertility of a five-year period, $b/5$ is shown instead. If we express the average fertility rate of a female who cannot take childcare leave as f_0 and that of one who can as f_1, the odds ratio is:

$$\exp(b) = \frac{f_1}{1-f_1} \Big/ \frac{f_0}{1-f_0}.$$

If the proportion of women who can take childcare leave is expressed as p, then the TFR can be written as follows:

$$TFR = 35\ \{(1-p)f_0 + pf_1\}.$$

The multiplier 35 comes from the length of the reproductive period. The expression above provides the following quadratic equation for f_0.

$$(1-p)\left(1-e^{-b}\right)f_0^2 + \left\{p + (1-p)e^{-b} - \frac{TFR}{35}\left(1-e^{-b}\right)\right\}f_0 - \frac{TFR}{35}e^{-b} = 0.$$

Although the expression is a little messy, it is possible to determine the value of f_0, if one were to provide an adequate value for each parameter. In Table 14, it is assumed that the TFR = 1.39 and $p = 0.167$. If there were no childcare leave provision in Japan, the TFR would be lower than it is today. The hypothetical TFR in the table is the value when $p = 0$. The table shows that the contribution of childcare leave is minor, contributing at most a TFR increase by 0.0531.

Table 14 Estimated effects of childcare leave in Japan

Literature	Suruga and Nishimoto (2002)	Shigeno and Matsuura (2003)	Yamaguchi (2005)	Suruga and Chang (2003)
b	0.0231	0.1244[a]	0.1886[a]	0.22298
$\exp(b)$	1.0234	1.1325	1.2076	1.2498
Fertility without leave (f_0)	0.0396	0.0389	0.0384	0.0382
Fertility with leave (f_1)	0.0405	0.0438	0.0461	0.0473
Current TFR	1.39	1.39	1.39	1.39
Hypothetical TFR[b]	1.3848	1.3612	1.3455	1.3369
Difference	−0.0052	−0.0288	−0.0445	−0.0531

[a] $b/5$

[b] TFR when nobody can take childcare leave

4.2.4 Childcare Services

Improving compatibility between female labor force participation and childrearing has been the primary political goal of the Japanese government. The Angel Plan announced in 1994 had "support for simultaneous child rearing and work" at the top of its list. In accordance with this directive, a major revision was made in 1997 to the Child Welfare Law, whereupon the public daycare service changed from a municipality assignment system (administrative measures) to a system that allows parents to select their preferred daycare center.

The New Angel Plan in 1999 sustained an emphasis on compatibility. The cabinet adopted in July 2001 a "Zero Waiting List for Daycare Program" as a political goal. As shown in Fig. 18, until 2007, the government's efforts were successful in reducing the number of children in waiting list. However, the demand for childcare, especially that for young children aged 1 and 2 years, sharply increased as of 2008, probably due to the subprime loan crisis. Thus, further efforts are required in this area.

4.2.5 Governmental Expenditure

In August 2012, the Act for the Total Reform of Tax and Social Security passed in Japan's Upper House. According to that act, the consumption tax rate would be raised from 5 to 8 % in April 2014, and to 10 % in October 2015. Three parties (i.e., DPJ, LDP, and NKP) agreed to direct JPY 2.7 trillion of the resulting revenue increase into the areas of family and social security. While JPY 2 trillion will be spent on the elderly people, the remaining JPY 0.7 trillion will be spent on children. Since governmental spending on children in 2012 is estimated to have totaled JPY 4.8 trillion (NIPSSR 2013), the spending of JPY 0.7 trillion implies a 14.6 % increase.

As seen in Table 15, in 2008, Japan spent 0.24 % of its GDP on childcare services. Even if this figure were increased by 14.6 %, the new figure of 0.28 % would not significantly change Japan's ranking.

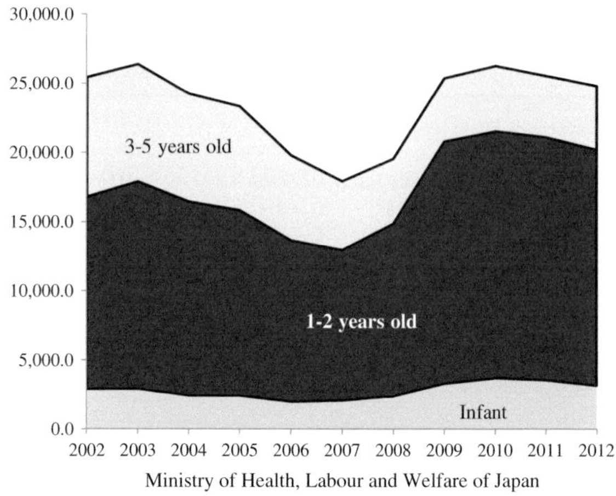

Fig. 18 Number of children in waiting list

Table 15 Public expenditure of childcare services (2008)

Country	% of GDP	Country	% of GDP
Denmark	0.85	Iceland	0.18
Finland	0.70	Italy	0.15
Norway	0.67	Czech Republic	0.12
Sweden	0.64	Canada	0.12
United Kingdom	0.44	Hungary	0.10
France	0.37	New Zealand	0.09
Luxembourg	0.36	Israel	0.09
Netherlands	0.34	Mexico	0.09
Belgium	0.24	Slovak Republic	0.08
Korea	0.24	United States	0.07
Japan	0.24	Germany	0.06
Australia	0.19		

OECD, *Economic Policy Reforms* 2012

4.3 Fertility Policy of Korea

Population policy in Korea can be divided into three time periods: the anti-natal period (1962–1996), the neutral period (1996–2004), and the pro-natal period (since 2004) (Choi Eun-Young et al. 2005). When the Park Chung-Hee government compiled the First Five-Year Plan for the National Economy (1962–1966), the policy planners were anxious about the negative impact of rapid population growth on the economy. The government launched a powerful family planning campaign to reduce the population growth rate to 2 % by 1971. Although the growth rate dropped below 2 % around 1970, the government's anti-natal program persisted. During the 1970s, tax relief was limited up to the second child, housing advantages were given to the acceptors of sterilization, and various contraceptive methods were subsidized. In spite of these interventions, the TFR in 1980 was as high as 2.83. The Chun Doo-Hwan government decided to expand the anti-natal campaign. Korea finally reached the replacement level in 1984.

Under the condition of below-replacement fertility and in response to agreements made during the International Conference on Population and Development in Cairo in 1994, the Noh Tae-Woo government decided in 1996 to abolish anti-natal population policy. During the neutral period in 1996–2004, the government's population policy sought to maintain status-quo fertility rates, improve mortality and morbidity rates, and normalize regional distribution. However, the TFR continued to decline and reached 1.47 in 1998 and 1.30 in 2001. While the Japanese government shifted to a pro-natal policy in response to its TFR of 1.57, the Kim Dae-Jung government (1998–2003) showed no reaction to having a TFR lower than 1.5. First, the government was busy in coping with the financial crisis in 1997. Second, as the anti-natal campaign had lasted for more than 30 years, Korean society found it difficult to reverse its attitudes toward fertility. It was when Korea's TFR fell as low as 1.17 in 2002 that the Noh Mu-Hyeon government took steps toward pro-natal intervention.

In 2004, the government launched the Presidential Committee on Aging and Future Society to compile new population policies. After a long discussion with representatives of business leaders, labor unions, activists, and feminists, the government action program "Saeromaji Plan 2010" was finally announced in 2006. This was an integrated policy package for the 2006–2010 period and its purpose was to help Korea to cope with low fertility and population aging. The fertility-oriented portion of the plan included various pro-natal measures, such as supporting daycare costs, rewarding large family through preferential taxation and housing benefits, improving childcare services, expanding maternity and childcare leaves, assisting in mothers' employment, and reinforcing family values.

In 2010, the Lee Myung-Bak government publicized the second-round package of population policies constituting the "Saeromaji Plan 2015," for the 2011–2015 period. As with the first package, the fertility-oriented part included various measures for improving compatibility between work and family, subsidizing the cost of childrearing, and ensuring the healthy development of children. The government document proposed such measures as expanding maternity-leave and childcare-leave programs, promoting flexible working conditions among government workers, and subsidizing maternity care, infertility treatments, and daycare services, among other things.

4.4 Fertility Policy of Taiwan

It seems that Korea and Taiwan share a common time-table in terms of economic and political developments. Rapid economic growth in the 1970s and 1980s produced the so-called Four Asian Dragons, with Hong Kong and Singapore. The democratization of Korea and Taiwan took place almost simultaneously, in 1987. Their transitions in population policy were also very close in time. While Korea launched the government family planning program in 1962, Taiwan started in 1964 (Ministry of Interior 2011). Korea abolished its anti-natal policy in 1996, and Taiwan abolished in 1992 (Lee Meilin 2009a; Chen Hsiao-Hung 2009). Government documents announcing the transition to a pro-natal policy were published in 2006 and 2008 in Korea and Taiwan, respectively.

Taiwan's Ministry of the Interior planned to publish the White Book of Population Policy including pro-natal policy measures in 2005. However, feminist and ecologist groups protested the policy transition, emphasizing Taiwan's overpopulation. As the result, the outline of the population policy, agreed upon in June 2006, included such principles as the promotion of reproductive health, improvements in the safety net, and environmental protection. It was also agreed that the White Book would constitute three distinct parts: child policy, elderly policy and immigration policy. Since its relationship with mainland China is the most sensitive political issue, there was a long discussion regarding immigration policy, which was closely related to the national defense issue. The White Book of Population Policy was finally published in March 2008. The fertility-oriented portion discussed various measures, such as daycare services, child allowance, work-life-balance, maternity leave, and childcare leave.

Despite these similarities, there was a sharp contrast between Korea and Taiwan concerning with respect to the role of formal education. The original document of the Saeromaji Plan 2010 stated that formal education should emphasize the value of marriage and the family, and should teach the happiness that comes with having and raising children. While this conservative tone seems to deny the life-style of remaining single or childless, Korean liberals or feminists agreed upon the document.

On the other hand, the section on "family values" in Taiwanese White Book was dominated by feministic values. It stated that traditional gender roles should be denied, and that the formal education system should be gender-neutral so that both boys and girls can learn about domestic work. The White Book blamed the persistent gender role as the cause of the recent nuptiality decline. Such feministic tone in this government document may correspond to the stronger political power of feminists and the higher gender equity in the formal sector in Taiwan, compared to Japan or Korea. On the other hand, the anxiety expressed within the document may correspond to Taiwan's lower gender equity within the family.

4.5 Fertility Policy of China

Political leaders in China started to be anxious by the early 1970s about the country's rapid population growth. Following ideological conflicts that occurred during the Cultural Revolution, the "one-child policy" was finally enforced in 1979. Couples in some areas can have a second child, in line with those areas' annual birth plans. Couples who break family planning regulations are fined (Hardee-Cleaveland and Bannister 1988; Chu and Yu 2010). In the late 1990s, 35.4 % of the Chinese population lived in areas with a strict one-child policy;

53.6 % lived in areas with a 1.5-children policy, where couples were allowed to have a second child, if the first child is a girl (Gu 2009).

Korea abandoned its anti-natal policy 12 years after below-replacement fertility was achieved, and Taiwan abandoned it after 8 years. However, China continues to sustain anti-natal policy, in spite of it having been at the below-replacement level for a considerable length of time. According to news articles, many experts have proposed banning the one-child policy. However, the former National Population and Family Planning Commission repeated that the policy will be firmly maintained during the Twelfth Guideline period (2011–2015). In March 2013, the former National Population and Family Planning Commission and the former Ministry of Health were integrated to form the National Health and Family Planning Commission. In November 2013, there was a relaxation of policy that a couple can have a second child if either spouse has no siblings. However, fertility policy of China is still quite anti-natal.

Japan shifted to a pro-natal policy in the early 1990s, more than a decade before the population actually started to decline, around 2010. According to the UNPD (2013), the population of Korea will start to decline in 2035–2040 and that of Taiwan in 2025–2030. According to official projections, that start of population decline will initiate in 2030–2035 in Korea and 2020–2025 in Taiwan (National Statistics Office 2011; Council for Economic Planning and Development 2010). In any case, Korea and Taiwan accomplished the transition to a pro-natal policy long before its population decline. While the UNPD (2013) predicts that the population of China will start to decline in 2030–2035, even the abolition of its anti-natal policy—not to mention the adoption of pro-natal policy—has not yet taken place. In China, the most populous nation in the world, the fear of overpopulation is so serious that a pro-natal policy may not be adopted until its population actually starts to decline. It is even possible that anti-natal policy is preserved until the momentum of population growth abates.

4.6 Conclusion

Practically all the policy methods to increase fertility were already implemented by either France or communist Eastern Europe during the twentieth century. They include baby bonuses, family allowances, paid maternity and parental leave, leave to care for sick children, tax relief for parents, care facilities for young children, flexible work arrangements, guarantees of retained promotion rights, labor force re-entry training programs, housing benefits, and educational supplements (Caldwell 2006). However, as the results of the quantitative evaluation of Japan in this section suggest, such pro-natal interventions have had little impact on increasing fertility. The difference in TFR caused by such a policy measure is always lower than 0.1, and sometimes even lower than 0.01.

One may think that the recovery of the TFR after 2005 in Japan and Korea and after 2010 in Taiwan has been the result of policy intervention. However, all countries that once suffered from lowest-low fertility have witnessed some recovery of their TFR values (Goldstein et al. 2009). The recovery in Eastern Asia could be seen as a natural response, and the role of policy intervention has not necessarily been significant. Considering the symbolic meaning of policy, however, a government still needs to make efforts to increase fertility, despite there being no "magic bullet". As McDonald (2002) writes, what is required of the government is the clear and simple message that "society will support you, if you have children." When the people believe that they will receive sufficient support, policy measures will start bringing about the desired effects.

5 Demography of Population Aging in Japan and Eastern Asia

5.1 Introduction

This section discusses population aging in Japan and Eastern Asia. The definitions used here with regard of three age groups are conventional: "child" refers to individuals aged under 15, "working-age" to those aged 15–64, and "elderly" to those aged 65 and over. As of the year 2010, Japan is the most aged country in the world. This condition was brought about by the combination of below-replacement fertility and one of the lowest mortality rates in the world, both since the mid-1970s. This also suggests the importance of mortality in population aging, even though the effect of fertility is more direct.

Population aging begins as soon as fertility starts to decline. However, because the percentage of working-age population grows more quickly than that of the elderly population, the total dependency ratio (i.e., children and elderly populations divided by the working-age population) declines for several decades. This decrease in net consumers relative to net producers is referred to as a "demographic bonus" or "demographic gift" (Mason 2001), or a "demographic window of opportunity" (Lee 2007). In any case, such change is supposed to promote economic development by increasing savings and investments and bringing about higher educational attainment. In Japan, this situation ended in the 1990s; presently, Japan has a "demographic debt" or "demographic onus," in which the dependency ratio grows continuously.

Considering the recent drastic fertility decline in Korea and Taiwan, these countries will quickly catch up with Japan in terms of population aging. It is also possible that Korea and Taiwan exceeds Japan in such indices as median age, the percentage of the elderly, or the elderly dependency ratio. Although Korea, Taiwan, and China are still enjoying a so-called demographic bonus, it is predicted that their total dependency ratios will start to increase soon. The decrease in working-age population and that of the total population are also expected within a decade or two. This section presents a simple stylized model to capture the effect of fertility decline on the magnitude and length of demographic bonus and the initiation of population decline.

5.2 Population Aging in Japan

5.2.1 Percentage of the Elderly and Average Ages

The percentage of the elderly in Japan was as low as 4.9 % in 1950. As shown in Fig. 19, the percentage rose sharply as fertility dropped drastically in the 1950s. Note that figures in this section are not based on UNPD (2013) but on Japanese census data, as well as the medium fertility and mortality variant in NIPSSR (2012a). The increase in this percentage has accelerated, but is predicted to slow down from the year 2015. In 2010–2015, the postwar baby boom cohort born in the late 1940s will be crossing the boundary of 65. After the cohort crosses the boundary of 75 in 2020–2015, there will remain little momentum for the population aged 65–74. Thus, the rise in percentage will mainly take place among individuals aged 75 and over. Although the change will slow down after 2015, the percentage of the elderly will increase from 23.0 % in 2010 to 31.6 % in 2030 and 39.9 % in 2060. The percentage of those aged 75 and over will also increase from 11.1 % in 2010 to 19.5 % in 2030 and 26.9 % in 2060. Thus, the percentage of those aged 75 years and older within the elderly population will grow from 48.1 % in 2010 to 61.8 % in 2030 and 67.4 % in 2060.

While the trajectory of the mean and median ages shows little acceleration as seen in the percentage of the elderly, the projection results of these measures suggest that there will be a slowing down in the future (Fig. 20). When the population was young, the mean age was higher than the median age, because the former tends to be influenced by high age values among a relatively small number of the elderly population. Thus, in 1950, the mean age was 26.6 and the median was 22.3. The difference narrowed in the course of population aging. In fact, in 2010, both the mean and median ages were 45.0 years. It is expected that the mean age will be lower than the median age in the future. In 2060, while the mean age of Japan's population is predicted to be 57.3 years, the median age is predicted to be 54.6 years. Because the medium fertility and mortality variant of NIPSSR (2012a) assumes a lower fertility level than UNPD (2013), the NIPSSR projected median age is higher than the UNPD projection of 53.3 years.

5.2.2 Dependency Ratios

Figure 21 shows the child dependency ratio, defined as the ratio of children to the working-age population, and the elderly dependency ratio, defined as the ratio of the elderly to the working-age population. The sum of these two ratios is the total dependency ratio. While Japan enjoyed a demographic bonus until 1990, the rapid aging of the population started to increase the total dependency ratio. According to

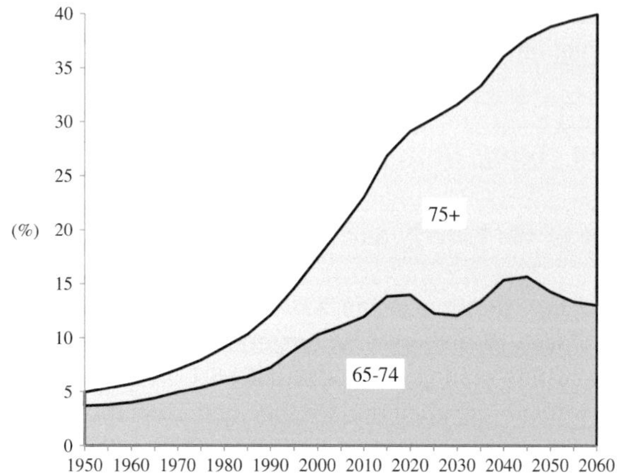

Fig. 19 Percentage of elderly population in Japan. NIPSSR (2013)

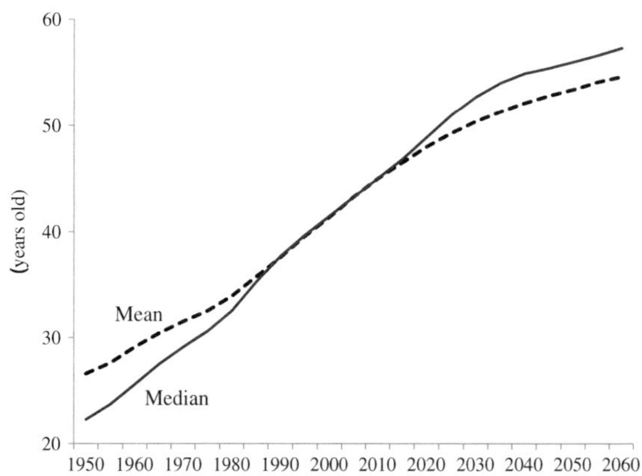

Fig. 20 Mean and median ages of population in Japan. NIPSSR (2013)

NIPSSR (2012b), Japan's elderly dependency ratio of 36.1 % in 2010 will swiftly reach 54.4 % in 2030 and 78.4 % in 2060. The total dependency ratio of 2060 implies that there will be 96.3 net consumers for 100 net producers, compared with 56.7 net consumers in 2010.

While total dependency ratios are easily obtained and can be compared among countries, the assumptions that all working-age individuals are net producers and all children and elderly individuals are net consumers are too simplistic. The best alternative is the "support ratio" used in National Transfer Account studies (Lee 2007; Mason and Lee 2012). However, per-capita income and consumption by age are difficult to obtain and project. Instead, what is attempted here is the calculation of the ratio of non-laborers to laborers, using census and existing projections.

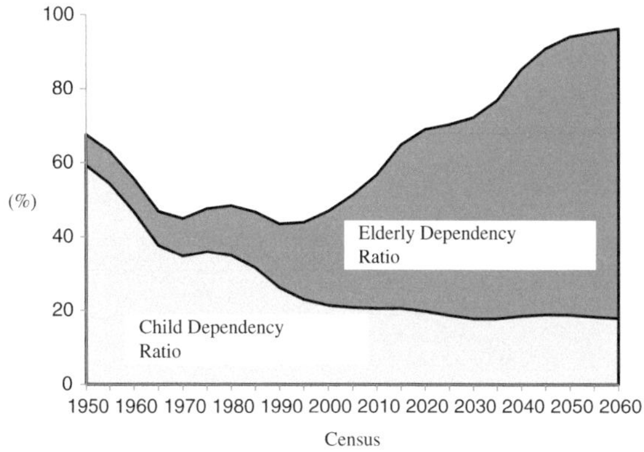

Fig. 21 Dependency ratios in Japan. NIPSSR (2013)

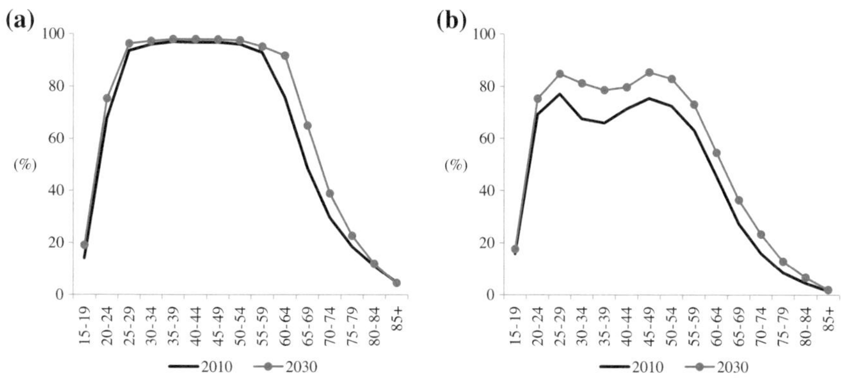

Fig. 22 Labor force participation rate (JILPT 2013, scenario C). **a** male, **b** female

The Japan Institute for Labour Policy and Training conducted projections of labor force participation, using three scenarios. Scenario A assumes that there will be practically no economic growth until 2030, and scenario C assumes that Japan's economy will grow at a 2 % annual growth rate. Scenario B, meanwhile, is the medium variant, and it assumes a 1 % annual economic growth. Figure 22 shows the projected change in labor force participation rates by age and sex in line with scenario C. Increases by more than 5 % points are expected for men aged 60–74 and women aged 25–74. Projected changes are smaller in scenario B and almost invisible in scenario A. All three scenarios assume that the M-shaped pattern for women will be sustained.

These projected labor force participation rates were applied to the projected population, to obtain non-labor/labor ratios by scenario. Figure 23 shows the results, along with total dependency ratios. The non-labor/labor ratio will increase from 54.0 % in 2010 to 69.4 % in 2030, if there is no significant change in labor force participation as scenario A assumes. However, the pressure of population

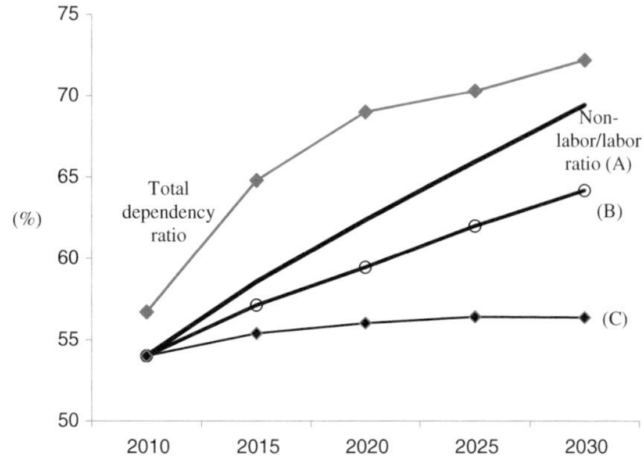

Fig. 23 Dependency ratio and non-labor/labor ratios. NIPSSR (2012b), JILPT (2013)

aging will be mostly compensated, if the increase in labor force participation that is projected in Scenario C (and as shown in Fig. 22) actually happens. The increase in the total dependency ratio is predicted to increase 15.5 % points, from 56.7 % in 2010 to 72.2 % in 2030. It is likely that a part of that increase will be compensated by the increase in labor force participation, although the degree depends on the economic conditions.

5.2.3 Japan: The Most Aged Country

This section examines the ranking of population aging based on UNPD (2013). As Table 16 confirms, in 2010, Japan is the most aged country. Twenty-four countries appear in this table. While Spain, France, Hungary, and the United Kingdom are not in the top 20 with respect to median age, the Channel Islands, Hong Kong, the Netherlands, and Martinique are not in the top 20 with respect to the percentage of elderly and the elderly dependency ratio. The ranking of the percentage of elderly and that of the elderly dependency ratio are very similar, while that of the median age is somewhat different from the other two.

According to Table 17, since 2005, Japan has been showing the highest percentage of elderly and the highest elderly dependency ratio. The highest median age in Japan was established earlier, in 1995. The table also shows the rank of Japan in terms of TFR and life expectancy at birth (both sexes combined) for each five-year period, as well as the rank in terms of the un-weighted average for 12 periods in 1950–2010. In fact, Japan had one of the lowest TFR values in 1955–1970, when many Western developed countries were experiencing postwar baby boom. At that time, only Latvia, Estonia, Hungary, Romania and what is now the Czech Republic had TFR values lower than Japan's. Japan's ranking fell after the second demographic transition took place among Western countries. Japan's life expectancy at birth quickly caught up to those of Western countries, and Japan has been showing

Table 16 Rankings of population aging in 2010

Percent of elderly 65+ (%)			Elderly dependency ratio (%)			Median age (years old)		
Rank	Country		Rank	Country		Rank	Country	
1.	Japan	22.96	1.	Japan	36.02	1.	Japan	44.86
2.	Germany	20.81	2.	Germany	31.63	2.	Germany	44.28
3.	Italy	20.29	3.	Italy	30.90	3.	Italy	43.29
4.	Greece	18.99	4.	Greece	28.56	4.	Bulgaria	42.44
5.	Latvia	18.37	5.	Sweden	27.88	5.	Finland	42.02
6.	Bulgaria	18.34	6.	Latvia	27.23	6.	Croatia	41.91
7.	Sweden	18.20	7.	Portugal	26.95	7.	Austria	41.83
8.	Portugal	18.01	8.	Bulgaria	26.83	8.	Greece	41.78
9.	Austria	17.83	9.	Austria	26.45	9.	Switzerland	41.57
10.	Croatia	17.54	10.	Croatia	26.11	10.	Slovenia	41.52
11.	Estonia	17.48	11.	Estonia	26.05	11.	Latvia	41.25
12.	Belgium	17.16	12.	Belgium	25.98	12.	Channel Islands	41.15
13.	Finland	17.13	13.	France	25.91	13.	Belgium	41.10
14.	Spain	17.10	14.	Finland	25.82	14.	Hong Kong	41.05
15.	Switzerland	16.91	15.	Denmark	25.49	15.	Portugal	41.04
16.	France	16.80	16.	United Kingdom	25.19	16.	Netherlands	40.84
17.	Hungary	16.72	17.	Spain	25.16	17.	Sweden	40.73
18.	Denmark	16.66	18.	Switzerland	24.85	18.	Denmark	40.59
19.	Slovenia	16.66	19.	Hungary	24.36	19.	Estonia	40.47
20.	United Kingdom	16.59	20.	Slovenia	24.03	20.	Martinique	40.32

Based on UNPD (2013)

Table 17 Rank of Japan

Year	Percent of elderly	Elderly dependency ratio	Median age	Period	Total fertility rate[a]	Life expectancy at birth
1950	75	78	75	1950–1955	29	37
1955	63	73	55	1955–1960	3	38
1960	55	67	43	1960–1965	5	35
1965	49	70	38	1965–1970	4	13
1970	45	62	31	1970–1975	21	8
1975	44	53	27	1975–1980	16	2
1980	44	45	21	1980–1985	16	1
1985	33	33	12	1985–1990	18	1
1990	23	27	3	1990–1995	9	1
1995	16	19	1	1995–2000	16	1
2000	3	4	1	2000–2005	19	1
2005	1	1	1	2005–2010	11	1
2010	1	1	1	1950–2010	6	7

Based on UNPD (2013)
[a] Rank from the lowest

Table 18 Un-weighted averages in 1950–2010

Rank	Country	Total fertility rate	Rank	Country	Life expectancy at birth
1.	Germany	1.7272	1.	Iceland	76.37
2.	Channel Islands	1.7639	2.	Sweden	76.16
3.	Latvia	1.7690	3.	Norway	75.84
4.	Luxembourg	1.7998	4.	Netherlands	75.67
5.	Italy	1.8276	5.	Switzerland	75.49
6.	Japan	1.8353	6.	Canada	74.87
7.	Switzerland	1.8370	7.	Japan	74.75
8.	Austria	1.8667	8.	Australia	74.74
9.	Hungary	1.8725	9.	Israel	74.50
10.	Estonia	1.8748	10.	Denmark	74.38
11.	Greece	1.8898	11.	France	74.24
12.	Slovenia	1.8944	12.	Hong Kong	74.13
13.	Bulgaria	1.9087	13.	Italy	74.13
14.	Czech Republic	1.9288	14.	Spain	74.06
15.	Ukraine	1.9309	15.	Cyprus	74.05
16.	Croatia	1.9310	16.	New Zealand	74.00
17.	Sweden	1.9344	17.	United Kingdom	74.00
18.	Belgium	1.9554	18.	Channel Islands	73.91
19.	Denmark	1.9738	19.	Belgium	73.51
20.	Russian Federation	1.9917	20.	Greece	73.45

Based on UNPD (2013)

the longest life expectancy since 1980. As for the entire 1950–2010 period, Japan had the sixth lowest TFR and the seventh longest life expectancy worldwide.

Table 18 lists the top 20 countries in terms of TFR and life expectancy at birth, for the entire 1950–2010 period. Japan and Switzerland are the only two countries listed in the lowest 10 countries in terms of both fertility and mortality. Among the five countries with lower TFR than Japan, Germany (21st), Latvia (54th), and Luxembourg (27th) do not appear in the top 20 in terms of life expectancy. Among the six countries with a life expectancy longer than Japan's, Iceland (50th), Norway (29th), the Netherlands (26th), and Canada (32nd) do not appear in the top 20 in terms of TFR.

In the following simple regression analysis, it is assumed that the un-weighted averages of TFRs, life expectancy values at birth, and net migration rates affect the proportion of the elderly or the median age in 2010. It is known that a mortality decline promotes population aging only when mortality is sufficiently low (Lee 1994). Thus, the square of life expectancy is included in the model. The natural log is taken of the proportion of the elderly, to preclude negative predictions. All the data from 201 countries and areas come from the UNPD (2013) (Table 19).

As expected, fertility decline promotes population aging. The effect of life expectancy is enhanced as longevity is prolonged. The net migration rate depresses the proportion of elderly but increases the median age. This implies that migrants tend to be younger than 65 but older than the median age of most countries. The

Table 19 Multiple regression of population aging

	Proportion of elderly (log)		Median age	
	Coef.	Std. Err	Coef.	Std. Err
Intercept	0.8331	0.5428	54.5658	5.8492**
Total fertility rate	−0.3385	0.0194**	−3.9245	0.2092**
Life expectancy	−0.0833	0.0196**	−0.4981	0.2112*
Life expectancy (squared)	0.0008	0.0002**	0.0055	0.0019**
Net migration rate	−0.0289	0.0021**	0.0717	0.0226**
R^2	0.9063		0.9247	

* $p < 0.05$, ** $p < 0.01$

predicted percentage of elderly for Japan is 17.7 %, and is highest in the world as in the observation. On the other hand, the predicted median age for Japan is 41.15 years old, which is fifth highest worldwide. Although the prediction does not necessarily reproduce the exact real-world ranking, the analysis confirms that Japan's very advanced population aging is the result of the combination of low fertility and low mortality.

5.3 Population Aging and Decline in Eastern Asia

According to UNPD (2013), Eastern Asian countries other than Japan still show relatively young age structures. In 2010, the percentage of the elderly in Korea was 11.1 % (55th). In Taiwan (labeled "other non-specified areas" in the UNPD documents), the figure was 10.7 % (56th), and in China, it was 8.4 % (70th). The median age in Korea was 37.8 (41st); in Taiwan, 37.1 (45th); and in China, 34.6 (59th). However, Korea's and Taiwan's rapid fertility decline to a level lower than that of Japan will supposedly bring about drastic population aging. As shown in Fig. 24, in 2060, the percentage of the elderly in these two countries is predicted to overcome that of Japan. On the other hand, the percentage in China is projected to stay below 30 %, as its fertility and mortality rates are assumed to stay at a higher level than other three countries.

The situation is similar for the median age, although the increase is quite linear (Fig. 25). The slopes of Korea and Taiwan are so steep that their median ages are projected to exceed that of Japan around 2050. China's slope is approximately the same as Japan's. As with the percentage of the elderly, the median age in China is also predicted to stay at a lower level than in the other three countries.

As mentioned, Japan has been in a "demographic onus" situation since 1990. According to the census results, the total dependency ratio of 66.9 % in 1947 was slightly lower than that in 1950 (67.5 %). Thus, it can be said that the continuous decline in total dependency ratio started in Japan around 1950, and that the demographic bonus lasted for 40 years. The starting points of Korea, Taiwan, and China can be determined from UNPD (2013) data. As shown in Fig. 26, the

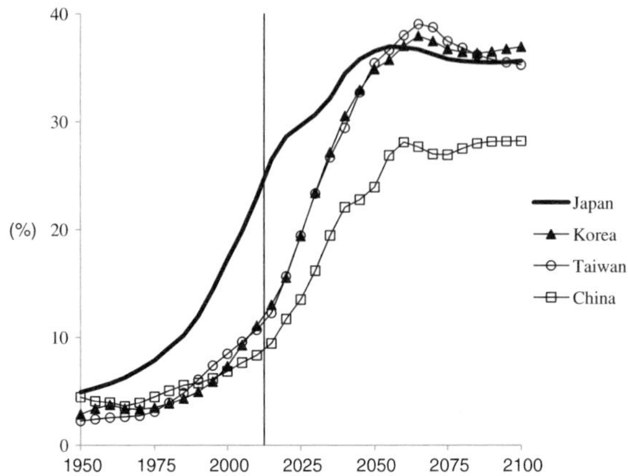

Fig. 24 Percentage of elderly in Eastern Asia. UNDP (2013)

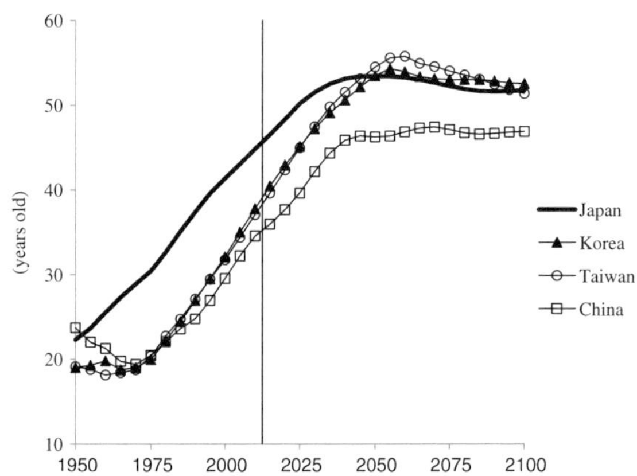

Fig. 25 Median age of population in Eastern Asia. UNDP (2013)

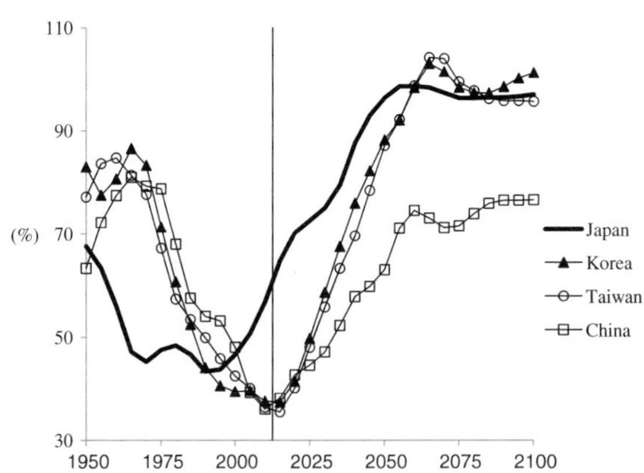

Fig. 26 Total dependency ratio in Eastern Asia. UNDP (2013)

demographic bonus began around 1960 in Taiwan and around 1965 in Korea and China. However, all three countries are approaching the turning point. It is projected that the total dependency ratio in China started to rise around 2010, and those of Korea and Taiwan will start to rise around 2015. Thus, for these three countries, the demographic bonus lasted longer than it did for Japan; 45 years for China (1965–2010), 50 years for Korea (1965–2015), and 55 years for Taiwan (1960–2015). In addition, the lowest total dependency ratio among each of the three countries is lower than that of Japan.

According to UNPD (2013), Japan's working-age population started to decline in the 1995–2000 period. In fact, the estimated working-age population of 87.161 million in 1996, according to the Statistics Bureau of Japan, was slightly smaller than that in the 1995 census (87.165 million). The working-age population continued to decline to 81.032 million in the 2010 census. The UNDP projection is that the working-age population in each of Korea, Taiwan and China will start to decline in the 2015–2020 period.

The turning point of the total population in Japan is more difficult to determine. NIPSSR (2002) projected that the first annual decline would take place in 2006–2007. However, the census population of 2005 was smaller than the population estimates for 2004. After this first annual decline, the estimated population increased in each of the 2005–2006, 2006–2007 and 2007–2008 periods. Experts suspected that there were serious undercounts in the 2005 census. This may be explained by the fact that the Japanese people were sensitive to providing personal information, as information security was a social issue at that time. While the estimated population declined in 2008–2009, the census population of 128.057 million in 2010 was larger than that estimated for 2009 (128.032). Estimates following the 2010 census have shown that there has been a constant decrease, to 127.799 million in 2011 and 127.515 million in 2012. Although the first decline occurred in 2004–2005, it is safer to state that Japan's turning point in population decline occurred in 2010–2011. According to UNPD (2013), the turning point is projected to be in 2025–2030 for Taiwan, in 2030–2035 for China, and in 2035–2040 for Korea.

Table 20 summarizes various turning points in the four countries. Although arrival at replacement level fertility is determined in terms of the five-year average values, vital statistics show that it was actually in 1956 in Japan (TFR of 2.22), in 1983 in Korea (TFR of 2.08), and in 1984 in Taiwan (TFR of 2.06). The child population can start to decline before the replacement level is achieved, although the growth rate of the number of births will converge to the intrinsic rate of natural increase in a long run. If fertility stays at the below-replacement level, the working-age population will start to decline, and finally the elderly population will start to decrease.

Some questions can be raised with regard to population aging and decline in Eastern Asia. Is there any mathematical reason for the median age to increase more linearly than the percentage of the elderly? Why are the total dependency ratios in Korea, Taiwan and China projected to continue to decline longer, and to a level lower than Japan's? What is the mathematical relationship between fertility

Table 20 Turning points in Eastern Asian populations

Turning points	Japan	Korea	Taiwan	China
	Period			
Replacement level	1955–1960	1985–1990	1985–1990	1990–1995
Total population decline	2010–2015	2035–2040	2025–2030	2030–2035
Child population decline	1955–1960	1975–1980	1970–1975	1975–1980
Working age population decline	1995–2000	2015–2020	2015–2020	2015–2020
Elderly population decline	2045–2050	2060–2065	2050–2055	2060–2065
	Demographic bonus			
Total dependency ratio decrease	1950	1965	1960	1965
Total dependency ratio increase	1990	2015	2015	2010
Duration	40	50	55	45
Minimum total dependency ratio	43.4	37.4	35.5	36.0
	Years after the replacement level			
Total population decline	55	50	40	40
Child population decline	0	−10	−15	−15
Working age population decline	40	30	30	25
End of Demographic Bonus	35	30	30	20
Elderly population decline	90	75	65	70

Based on UNPD (2013)

decline and each of the various turning points? The next section presents a very simple stylized model that can be used to discuss these points.

5.4 Stylized Linear Model of Population Aging

5.4.1 Definition of the Model

Assume that the initial population is expressed with a right triangle, whose base represents the maximum age ω and height is the number of births (or, the infant population of the exact age zero) B. A numerical example is $\omega = B = 100$ and the total population is $\omega B/2 = 5{,}000$. If B is expressed in thousands, a total population of 5 million is assumed. Let β be the lower age limit of the elderly population. If $\beta = 65$, the initial elderly population is $35^2/2 = 612.5$, and their percentage of the total population will be 12.25 %. This initial value is higher than that seen in the real world, where most countries start with a value lower than 7 %.

In the year t, it is assumed that the population younger than t is expressed with a straight line whose slope is c while the population older than t stays at the initial state (see Fig. 27). While Feeney and Mason (2001) presented a pentagon model, it is assumed here that the population is expressed with a quadrilateral. For population aging to take place, the slope c must be larger than $-B/\omega$; namely $-1 < c$ when $\omega = B = 100$. The intercept, or the infant population, in t is $B - (B/\omega + c)t$, which implies that the number of births decreases by $B/\omega + c$ every year. The population of exact age x in year t is:

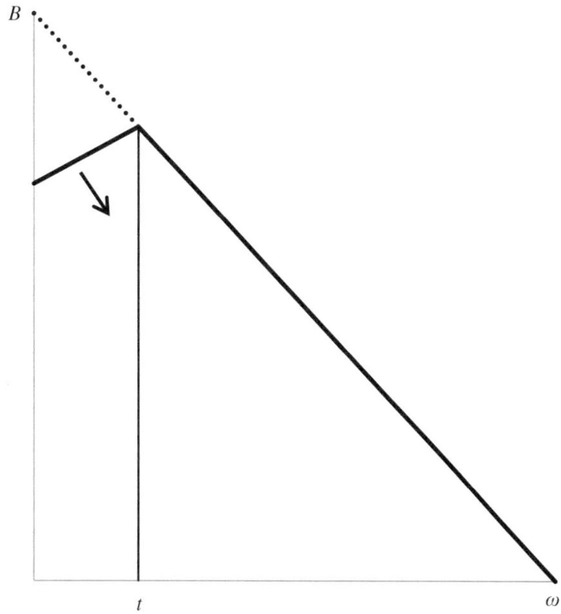

Fig. 27 Stylized linear model

$$P(x,t) = B - (\frac{B}{\omega} + c)t + cx, \quad 0 \le x < t, \tag{8}$$

$$P(x,t) = B - \frac{B}{\omega}x, \quad t \le x \le \omega. \tag{9}$$

This model is valid only until a negative population appears. If the slope c is positive, the infant population can be negative prior to the year ω. If $c = 1$, the model is valid for only 50 years. The slope c can be considered the tempo of fertility decline. The larger the slope, the more marked population aging will be. The total population in t is:

$$TP(t) = \frac{B\omega^2 - (B + \omega c)t^2}{2\omega}. \tag{10}$$

If $\omega = B=100$, then $TP(t) = 5000 - 0.5(1 + c)\ t^2$.

5.4.2 Percentage of the Elderly Population

The elderly population remains the same during $t < \beta$, being expressed with a right triangle with a base of $\omega - \beta$ and a height of $P(\beta, 0) = B - B\beta/\omega$. When $\beta \le t$, the elderly population is a sum of a right triangle with $\omega - t$ and $P(t, 0)$ and a trapezoid with $P(t, 0)$ and $P(\beta, t)$ as bases and $t - \beta$ as the height. After all, the proportion of the elderly in t is:

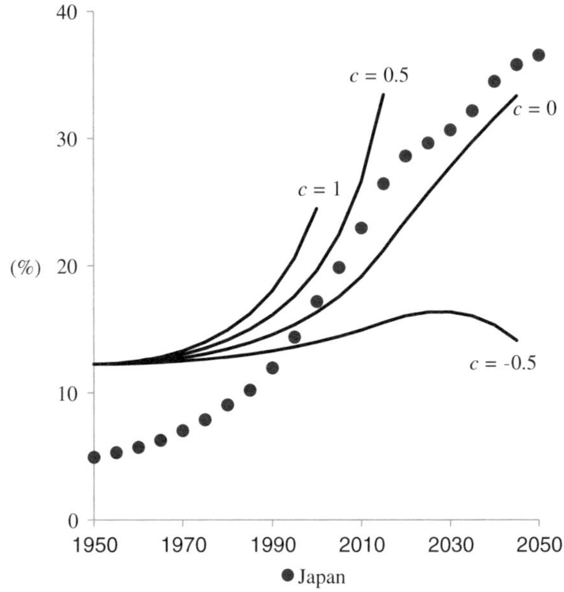

Fig. 28 Percentage of elderly

$$f_\beta(t) = \frac{(\omega - \beta)^2}{\omega^2 - (1 + \omega c/B)t^2}, \quad t<\beta, \tag{11}$$

$$f_\beta(t) = \frac{B(\omega - t)(t - 2\beta + \omega) - \omega c(t - \beta)^2}{B\omega^2 - (B + \omega c)t^2}, \quad \beta \leq t. \tag{12}$$

It can be shown that when $\omega = B = 100$, $f_{65}(t)$ increases monotonously during $t < \beta$. As shown in Fig. 28, $f_{65}(t)$ can decline after $\beta \leq t$ if $c < 0$. The increase in $f_{65}(t)$ is accelerated if $0 < c$. Given the constant initial value of 12.25 %, it is impossible to approximate the observed trajectory.

5.4.3 Median Age

The initial median age is also constant, at $x_M(0) = \omega - \omega/\sqrt{2}$, or 29.29 years old when $\omega = B = 100$. To obtain the median age in $t > 0$, it is necessary to determine the year τ_M when τ_M is also the median age in that year.

$$\tau_M = \frac{2 - \sqrt{1 - \omega c/B}}{3 + \omega c/B}\omega. \tag{13}$$

It can be shown that τ_M is an increasing function of c. If $c = 0$, $\tau_M = 33.3$ years. The median age $x_M(t)$ is obtained according to t and c.

Fig. 29 Median age

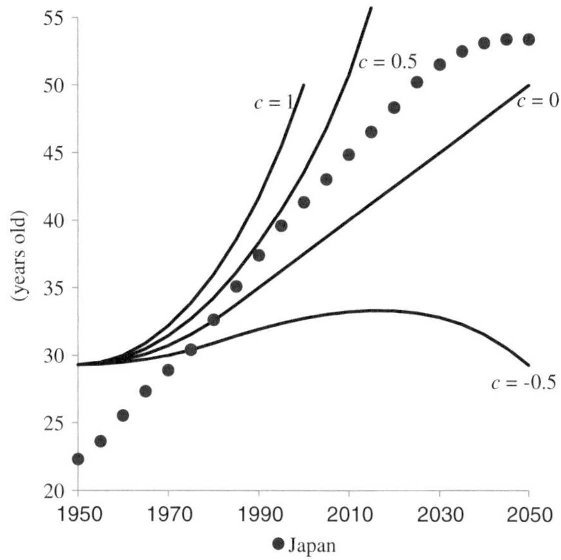

$$x_M(t) = \omega - \sqrt{\frac{\omega}{B} TP(t)} = \omega - \sqrt{\frac{\omega^2 - (1 + \omega c/B)t^2}{2}}, \quad t < \tau_M, \tag{14}$$

$$x_M(t) = \frac{-P(0,t) + \sqrt{P(0,t)^2 + c\ TP(t)}}{c}, \quad \tau_M \leq t,\ c \neq 0, \tag{15}$$

$$x_M(t) = \frac{\omega + t}{4}, \quad \tau_M \leq t,\ c = 0. \tag{16}$$

Unlike the proportion of the elderly, the median age can change quite linearly, especially when c approximates 0. On the other hand, the median age can decrease if $c < 0$, as with the proportion of the elderly. Again, it is impossible to approximate the observed trajectory, given the constant initial value (Fig. 29).

5.4.4 Total Dependency Ratio

Let α be the boundary between the child and working-age populations. If the child population is written $C(t)$, the working-age population $W(t)$, and the elderly population $E(t)$, the populations by age group are:

$$C(t) = \frac{B\alpha(2\omega - \alpha)}{2\omega} - \left(\frac{B}{2\omega} + \frac{c}{2}\right)t^2, \quad 0 \leq t < \alpha, \tag{17}$$

$$C(t) = B\alpha + \frac{c\alpha^2}{2} - \alpha\frac{B + \omega c}{\omega}t, \quad \alpha \leq t, \tag{18}$$

$$W(t) = W(0) = \frac{B(\beta - \alpha)(2\omega - \alpha - \beta)}{2\omega}, \quad 0 \le t < \alpha, \tag{19}$$

$$W(t) = B(\beta - \alpha) - \frac{B\beta^2}{2\omega} - \frac{\alpha^2 c}{2} + \frac{\alpha(B + \omega c)}{\omega} t - \frac{B + \omega c}{2\omega} t^2, \quad \alpha \le t < \beta, \tag{20}$$

$$W(t) = B(\beta - \alpha) - \frac{(\beta^2 - \alpha^2)c}{2} - \frac{(\beta - \alpha)(B + \omega c)}{\omega} t, \quad \beta \le t, \tag{21}$$

$$E(t) = E(0) = \frac{B(\omega - \beta)^2}{2\omega}, \quad 0 \le t < \beta, \tag{22}$$

$$E(t) = \frac{B(\omega - t)(t - 2\beta + \omega) - \beta c(t - \beta)^2}{2\omega}, \quad \beta \le t. \tag{23}$$

When $\omega = B = 100$, the initial populations are $C(0) = 1387.5$, $W(0) = 3000$, $E(0) = 612.5$, and the initial value of total dependency ratio is 66.7 %. This percentage happens to approximate the total dependency ratio of 67.6 % in Japan in 1950 (Fig. 30). However, the model cannot emulate the rapid decline in the ratio. The model ratio can go down to 40.85 %, which is lower than the observed bottom for Japan (43.40 % in 1990). The model stops there, however, because it is at this point that the negative infant population appears. For the turning point when the ratio starts to increase to be included within the limits of the model, it is necessary that $c < 11760/12240 = 0.9608$. This implies that the valid turning point τ_D is 51 years or less.

It is assumed here that the turning point τ_D is between α and β ($\alpha \le \tau_D < \beta$). In this case, the total dependency ratio is obtained from (18), (20), and (22). Especially when $\omega = B = 100$, the turning point τ_D is the smaller root of $3(1 + c)t^2 - 5(169 + 9c)t + 3000 = 0$:

$$\tau_D = \frac{5\left(169 + 9c - \sqrt{81c^2 - 11358c + 14161}\right)}{6(1 + c)}. \tag{24}$$

It can be shown that the more rapidly fertility decline takes place, the longer the demographic bonus lasts. As shown in Fig. 31, the demographic bonus usually lasts for 40–50 years. In this stylized model, the magnitude of fertility decline is expressed by the slope c in Fig. 27 and the slope is held constant over time. Thus, it is implicitly assumed that fertility stays at a level that produces a linear change. It is also shown that a rapid fertility decline results in a lower total dependency ratio (Fig. 32). Although the minimum value of the total dependency ratio varies between 40 and 65 %, the values lower than 40 % that are predicted for Korea, Taiwan and China (see Table 20) cannot be produced through this model.

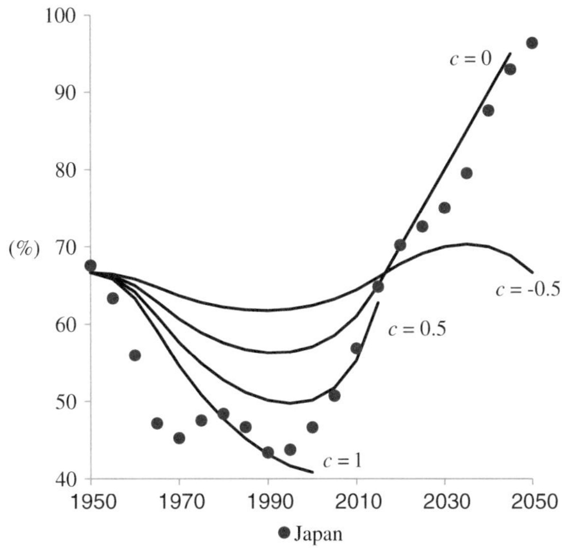

Fig. 30 Total dependency ratio

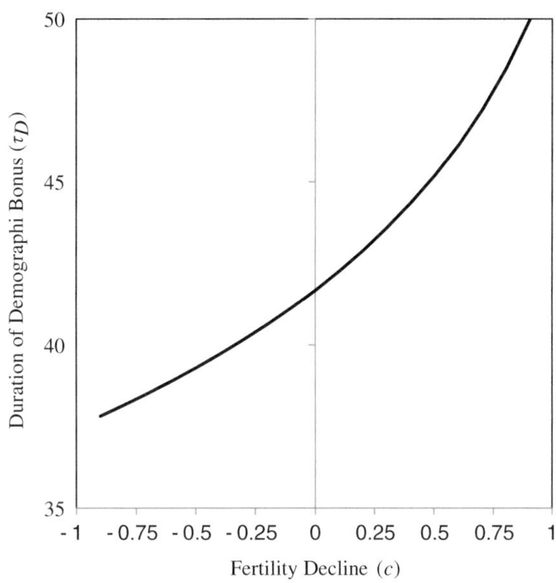

Fig. 31 Relationship between fertility decline and duration of demographic bonus

5.4.5 Momentum of Population Growth

It has been implicitly assumed thus far that the initial population was stationary and that the total population immediately starts to decline. To discuss the turning point at which the population starts to decline, it is necessary to assume that the initial population was stable and had a constant growth rate $r_0 > 0$. To preserve the

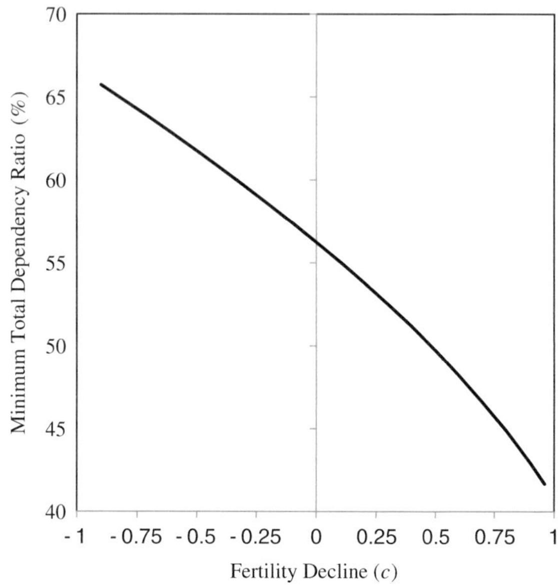

Fig. 32 Relationship between fertility decline and minimum dependency ratio

results obtained above, all the age-specific populations in a specific year should be multiplied by the same coefficient. Usually, $(1 + r_0)^t$ or $\exp(r_0\, t)$ is applied to achieve primary homogeneity. However, the following linear growth model is applied here for mathematical simplicity.

$$P_g(x,t) = (1 + r_0 t)\ P(x,t). \tag{25}$$

In this case, the total population is:

$$TP_g(t) = (1 + r_0 t)\ TP(t) = \frac{B\omega^2 + r_0 B\omega^2 t - (B + \omega c)t^2 - r_0(B + \omega c)t^3}{2\omega}. \tag{26}$$

Because the model discussed here makes use of a closed population lacking migration, the population growth rate is equivalent to the natural growth rate.

$$NGR(t) = \frac{TP'_g(t)}{TP_g(t)} = \frac{r_0 B\omega^2 - 2(B + \omega c)t - 3r_0(B + \omega c)t^2}{(1 + r_0 t)\{B\omega^2 - (B + \omega c)t^2\}}. \tag{27}$$

5.4.6 Decline of Total Population

Let τ_T be the time when the population growth rate in (27) turns negative. When $\omega = B = 100$, τ_T is the larger root of $3\ r_0(1 + c)t^2 + 2(1 + c)t - 1000r_0 = 0$.

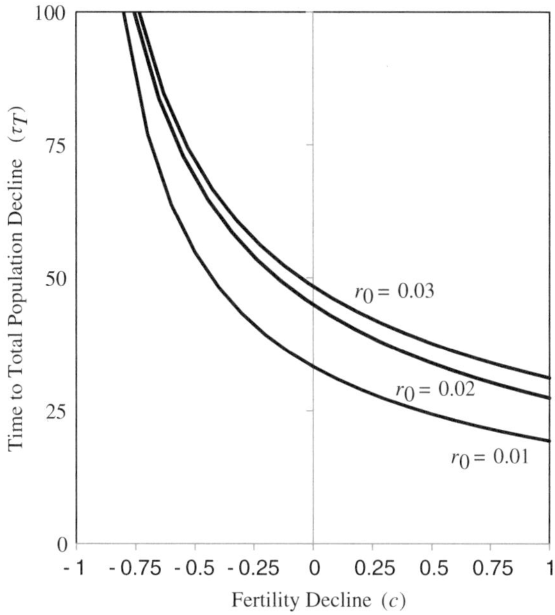

Fig. 33 Time to total population decline

$$\tau_T = -\frac{1}{3r_0} + \frac{\sqrt{(1+c)^2 + 30000\, r_0^2 (1+c)}}{3r_0(1+c)}. \tag{28}$$

As in Fig. 33, a rapid fertility decline (i.e., large c) results in an early beginning of decline in the total population. A rapid initial population growth (i.e., large r_0) lengthens the time until population decline. However, its impact diminishes when fertility decline was drastic. Although the model suggests that the total population can start to decline in fewer than 30 years following the arrival of below-replacement fertility, this is an unrealistically short timeframe. This is the limit of the model, assuming that the TFR suddenly "bottoms out" and stays at a certain level. It is difficult to determine the corresponding point of $t = 0$ within this model.

5.4.7 Decline of Population by Age Group

It is always assumed in this section that $\omega = B = 100$, $\alpha = 15$ and $\beta = 65$. Let τ_C be the time until the child population starts to decline. We need to determine whether or not τ_C occurs within 15 years.

$$\tau_C = -\frac{1}{3r_0} + \frac{\sqrt{(1+c)\left(1+c+8325\, r_0^2\right)}}{3r_0(1+c)}, \quad \tau_C < 15, \tag{29}$$

$$\tau_C = \frac{50 + 3.75\,c}{1 + c} - \frac{1}{2\,r_0}, \quad 15 \le \tau_C. \tag{30}$$

The condition for τ_C to occur earlier than 15 years is $(140\ r_0 - 2)/(45\ r_0 + 2) < c$. If r_0 were 1 %, even a negative c (i.e., $-0.24 < c$) could make the child population start to decline in fewer than 15 years. However, if the initial growth rate were 2 %, a larger c (i.e., $0.28 < c$) would be required to overcome the momentum of population growth within 15 years.

In this model, the working-age population always starts to decline after 15 years. The turning point τ_W is the lager root of $3\ r_0(1 + c)\ t^2 - 2(1 + c)(30\ r_0 - 1)\ t - 30(1 + c) - 75\ r_0(77 - 3c) = 0$.

$$\tau_W = \frac{30r_0 - 1}{3r_0} + \frac{\sqrt{(900\ r_0^2 + 30r_0 + 1)(1 + c)^2 + 225r_0^2(77 - 3c)(1 + c)}}{3r_0(1 + c)}. \tag{31}$$

For τ_W to occur sooner than 65 years, c should be larger than $-(1 + 30\ r_0)/(1 + 90\ r_0)$. If r_0 were 5 %, $-0.45 < c$ can make the working-age population start to decline earlier than in the 65th year. Although graphs are not shown, the effects of fertility decline (c) and initial population growth (r_0) are basically the same as those in Fig. 33. The decline of the elderly population occurs in the distant future, in 2045–2050 in Japan (see Table 20). Thus, the equation is not discussed here.

5.5 *Population Aging in Low Fertility Countries*

5.5.1 Low Fertility Countries

This section verifies the findings obtained above, through the use of UNPD (2013) projections. Here, "low fertility countries" are defined as those countries with below-replacement fertility in 2005–2010 and with a total population in 2010 greater than 1 million. Table 21 includes 64 low fertility countries in Eastern Asia (6 countries), South-eastern Asia (5), Eastern Europe (12), Northern Europe (9), Southern Europe (9), Western Europe (6), Northern America (2), Latin America and Caribbean (6) and others (9). For the 2005–2010 period, the TFR of Korea (1.228) is the third lowest, Taiwan (1.261) is fifth, and Japan (1.339) is 10th.

The highest and lowest TFR values by country after 1950 were searched. Because there is a secular trend in fertility decline, the lowest value always appears after the highest value. The "velocity of fertility decline" is simply the change in TFR divided by the timespan between the highest and lowest values. The most drastic fertility decline can be found in Hong Kong (0.127), followed by China (0.114), Korea (0.114), Singapore (0.097), and Latvia (0.096). Interestingly, the

Table 21 Fertility decline in low fertility countries

#.	Country	Velocity	#.	Country	Velocity
1.	Japan	0.034	33.	Portugal	0.037
2.	Korea	0.114	34.	Italy	0.043
3.	Taiwan	0.081	35.	Spain	0.066
4.	China	0.114	36.	Serbia	0.031
5.	Hong Kong	0.127	37.	Croatia	0.028
6.	DPR Korea	0.036	38.	Slovenia	0.027
7.	Singapore	0.097	39.	Greece	0.031
8.	Thailand	0.073	40.	Macedonia	0.040
9.	Viet Nam	0.081	41.	Albania	0.058
10.	Myanmar	0.055	42.	Germany	0.039
11.	Malaysia	0.050	43.	Austria	0.035
12.	Bosnia and Herzegovina	0.065	44.	Switzerland	0.030
13.	Slovakia	0.046	45.	Netherlands	0.083
14.	Hungary	0.028	46.	Belgium	0.044
15.	Poland	0.047	47.	France	0.037
16.	Romania	0.050	48.	Canada	0.053
17.	Ukraine	0.033	49.	USA	0.095
18.	Belarus	0.033	50.	Cuba	0.059
19.	Bulgaria	0.029	51.	Puerto Rico	0.052
20.	Czech Republic	0.033	52.	Trinidad and Tobago	0.071
21.	Russia	0.036	53.	Brazil	0.056
22.	Moldova	0.034	54.	Chile	0.053
23.	Georgia	0.028	55.	Costa Rica	0.085
24.	Lithuania	0.029	56.	Australia	0.037
25.	Latvia	0.096	57.	Cyprus	0.037
26.	Estonia	0.087	58.	Lebanon	0.066
27.	Finland	0.069	59.	Mauritius	0.085
28.	Denmark	0.058	60.	Armenia	0.055
29.	UK	0.029	61.	Iran	0.056
30.	Sweden	0.021	62.	UAE	0.067
31.	Norway	0.061	63.	Azerbaijan	0.048
32.	Ireland	0.072	64.	Tunisia	0.072

Based on UNDP (2013)

U.S. fertility decline (0.095) was sixth-fastest, because that country's minimum TFR appeared as early as 1975–1980. Taiwan's velocity (0.081) was 12th largest. On the other hand, the velocity in Japan (0.034) was very small, ranking 50th among 64 countries. If the exact annual values in the vital statistics are used, the maximum value after 1945 was 4.54 in 1947 and the minimum value was 1.26 in 2005. In this case, the velocity is $(4.54 - 1.26)/58 = 0.0566$; this ranks Japan at 25th. However, the result does not change the finding that the fertility decline in Japan was much slower than China, Korea, and Taiwan.

5.5.2 Tempo of Population Aging

It is assumed that a rapid fertility decline results in rapid population aging. The stylized linear model also shows that a large *c* gives rise to rapid increases in the percentage of the elderly and the median age. Such relations can be seen in 64 low fertility countries. The velocities of population aging were calculated in the same way as for fertility. The maximum values of the percentage of the elderly and the median age always appear after the minimum values. Thus, the difference between maximum and minimum is divided by the timespan.

The correlation between fertility decline and the increase in the percentage of the elderly (Fig. 34) is relatively weak. The unit of vertical axis is percentage points. Thus, low fertility countries are expected to experience annual increase of 0.1–0.4 points in the percentage of the elderly population. While population aging in Japan, Korea, and Taiwan is faster than predicted, that in China is slower. The main reason might be the difference in mortality decline, as mentioned above. Thus, while Korea and Taiwan will surpass Japan in terms of a faster fertility decline than Japan, China will not catch up with Japan in spite of China having a velocity of fertility decline equal to that of Korea.

The correlation between fertility decline and the rise in median age (Fig. 35) is stronger than that between fertility decline and the percentage of the elderly. Low fertility countries are expected to experience an annual increase in median age of 0.22 years on average. Again, the three Eastern Asian countries other than China are projected to experience faster increases that are occurring more quickly than predicted due to a faster-than average mortality decline. In fact, the assumed life expectancy at birth in 2095–2100 is highest in Korea (95.454), followed by Hong Kong (94.934), Japan (94.191), and Singapore (94.039). Among the low fertility countries, the assumed life expectancy at birth in Taiwan (90.262) is 25th, and China (85.348) is 47th.

5.5.3 Demographic Bonus

The stylized linear model suggests that a fast fertility decline results in a longer demographic bonus, and a lower total dependency ratio. Figure 36 confirms the latter relationship. Thus, it is natural that the lowest total dependency ratio in Japan is higher than that of Korea, Taiwan, and China, because fertility decline was slower in Japan. Although the United Arab Emirates is an extreme outlier in this graph, the reasons for this are outside the scope and they are not discussed here.

As for the duration of the demographic bonus, its starting point is not always self-evident. In each of the United Kingdom, Sweden, Norway and Belgium, the total dependency ratio has been increasing since 1950. Thus, the duration is unknown for these four countries. Even if the minimum ratio value were found after 1950, the ratio can temporarily rise before the continuous increase starts, as in the case of Japan (see Figs. 21 and 26). If "continuous decline for 10 years" were the criterion, the starting point of Japan's demographic bonus should be in 1980.

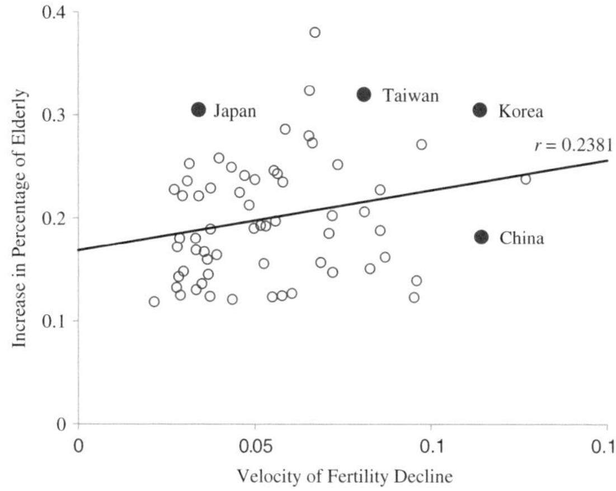

Fig. 34 Fertility decline and increase in percentage of elderly

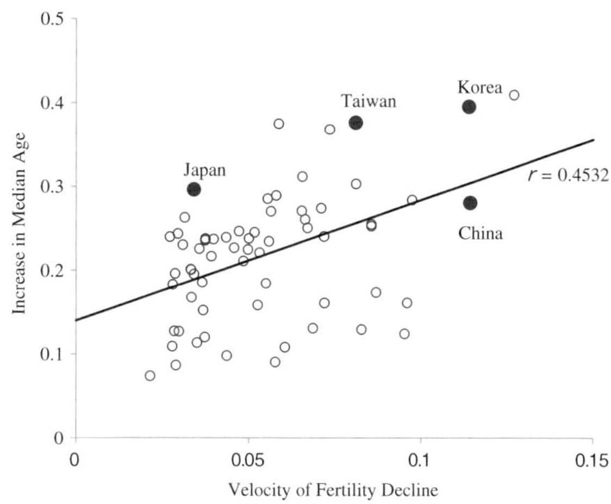

Fig. 35 Fertility decline and increase in median age

Thus, the starting point is defined here as that of a continuous decline over 15 years, or over three sequential five-year periods. For Japan, census results confirm that the starting point was 1950. In addition to Japan, the starting point of 1950 was pinpointed for Latvia (duration of 1950–2005), Estonia (1950–2005) and Cuba (1950–2015). Although the duration of the bonus for each of these countries is longer than that of Japan, there remains the possibility of underestimation. As shown in Table 22, the mean duration of the demographic bonus among 60 countries is 44.5 years and the correlation coefficient with the velocity of fertility decline is 0.2035. Thus, it is confirmed that a rapid fertility decline results in a long-term demographic bonus.

As shown in Table 20, the duration in China (45 years) is shorter than that of Korea (50 years) or Taiwan (55 years), in spite of its drastic fertility decline. The reason is that a small baby boom is predicted for China in 2010–2020. In the case of

Fig. 36 Fertility decline and minimum total dependency ratio

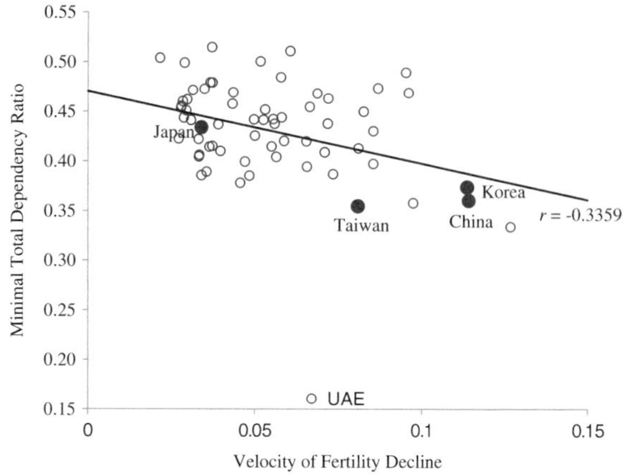

Table 22 Length to turning points and correlation with fertility decline

Length	Mean	Number of countries	Correlation with fertility decline
Duration of demographic bonus	44.5	60	0.2035
From replacement fertility			
To natural decrease	39.1	55	0.2161
To decline in total population	42.2	54	0.1750
To decline in working-age population	41.3	63	0.0153

Based on UNPD (2013)

Japan, a baby boom in the 1970s temporarily increased the total dependency ratio before it hit its lowest value in 1990. In China, the increase caused by the baby boom will be directly followed by an increase due to population aging. Thus, the demographic bonus in China is projected to be shortened by its initial age structure.

5.5.4 Population Decline

Table 22 summarizes the amounts of time to various turning points, as well as the correlation with the velocity of fertility decline. The duration of demographic bonus has already been discussed. The arrival at the replacement level is defined in terms of a series of three five-year periods of below-replacement fertility. In the same way, population decline is defined here in terms of three five-year periods of negative increase.

The stylized linear model suggests that a rapid fertility decline results in an early population decline. However, the correlation in low fertility countries does not support this relationship; rather, it indicates a positive correlation. The problem lies in how "arrival at replacement level" is defined. Some European countries experienced below-replacement fertility in the 1930s and a fertility decline started again after the postwar baby boom. For example, the natural growth rate of Germany has been negative since 1970–1975, and so the timespan there since below-replacement fertility is zero. The lack of fertility data before 1950 makes it difficult to capture the relationship between fertility decline and the start of population decrease.

In Eastern Asia, the time until population decrease in Japan (55 years, according to Table 20) is longer than that in Korea, Taiwan, and China, as the model suggests. On the other hand, the timespan of Korea (50 years) is longer than that of Taiwan (40 years), although fertility decline was more severe in Korea (see Table 21). Note that the population decline has not yet started; it is only *projected* for these countries. As mentioned, Korea and Taiwan arrived at below-replacement fertility in the early 1980s. The start to population decline in Korea (2035–2040) slower than that in Taiwan (2025–2030) depends on the assumption of UNPD (2013) with respect to fertility recovery. The recovery of TFR in Korea (1.52 in 2025–2030) is assumed to occur more rapidly than in Taiwan (1.35 in 2025–2030). However, the National Statistics Office of Korea (2011) assumes slower recovery, to 1.41 in 2030, and predicts that its total population will start to decline in 2030–2035. In this way, the timespan between below-replacement fertility and the decline in total population will depend not only on the velocity of fertility decline, but also on the speed of fertility recovery.

5.6 Conclusion

This section discussed the trajectory of population aging in Japan, while referring to data on the percentage of the elderly, mean or median age, and dependency ratios. It was also suggested that the increase in the non-labor/labor ratio may not occur as quickly as that of the total dependency ratio, if the pressure of population aging can be compensated to some extent by an increase in labor force participation rates. As for the position of Japan as the most aged country in the world, a simple regression analysis revealed that it was the combination of low fertility and low mortality that brought about this result.

A stylized linear model was presented to examine the impact of fertility decline not only on the percentage of the elderly or median age, but also on the total dependency ratio and the timing of population decline. The model suggested that a rapid fertility decline results in rapid population aging, a lower dependency ratio, a longer demographic bonus, and an earlier population decline. Most of these results were confirmed with low fertility countries in the UN projections.

Other eastern Asian countries than Japan experienced longer demographic bonus and lower consumer/producer ratios than Japan, thanks to more drastic fertility decline than Japan. This demographic window of opportunity may have supported the impressively compressed economic development of those countries. However, population aging after the window is closed will be so drastic that its negative impact will surpass that of Japan. There is the fear that too early population aging in certain countries (including China) will hit them before their economies are fully developed and mature. The governments of Eastern Asian countries (including Japan) have hoped that the traditional familial supports for the elderly can check increases in public costs relating to pensions and medical or long-term care. However, changes in family lives that induced a drastic fertility decline have also promoted acute changes in intergenerational relationships and living arrangements. Section 6 will discuss the political issue of the shift from familial to government support for the elderly.

6 Politics of Population Aging in Japan and Eastern Asia

6.1 Introduction

In the preindustrial period, the family was the unit of practically all activities, including economic production, consumption, child-care, training of young members and elderly-care. In the course of industrialization, the socialization of elderly-care started earlier than that of child-care. In Japan, universal public pension and health insurance programs were introduced in 1961. However, other Eastern Asian countries were much slower than Japan to introduce a universal pension program. China seems to have special difficulty in preserving for government workers what is left of the socialist pension system, while expanding a pension system into rural areas.

Unexpected and compressed population aging in unprepared cases constitute a serious political issue. In China, the sense of relative deprivation due to rapid population aging before becoming a developed country (*weifu xianlao*) can be seen in the journalism. When thus unprepared, a government may wish to rely on familial support for the elderly, to avoid crippling increases in the public cost of pension, medical treatment, and long-term care for the disabled elderly. However, a drastic fertility decline implies a drastic decline in family resources that can be directed toward the elderly. In Japan, the percentage of the elderly living with children has been in decline, probably due to the smaller number of children, the transition in family norms from the traditional stem family to the nuclear family, and the rising divorce rate. It is most likely that the same conditions are being experienced in other Eastern Asian countries. Thus, the role of public support becomes more and more important as the pressures of population aging increase.

6.2 Living Arrangements of the Elderly

6.2.1 Living Arrangements of the Elderly in Japan

Figure 37 shows the changes in living arrangements among the elderly people of Japan. Note that those living in institutional households are excluded from the denominator. The percentage of the elderly living with children declined from

Fig. 37 Living arrangements of elderly aged 65+ in Japan

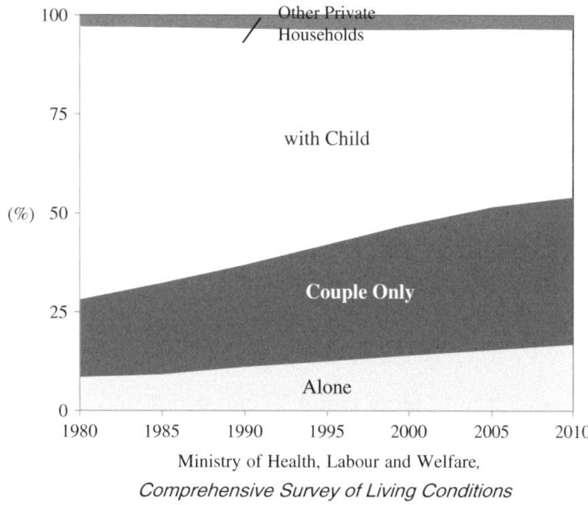

69.0 % in 1980 to 42.3 % in 2010. In the same period, the percentage living alone rose from 8.5 to 16.9 %, and that of those living only with a spouse rose from 19.6 to 37.2 %. It is likely that the fertility decline promoted this change by reducing the availability of children with whom they can coreside (Hirosima 1983, 1984). The literature suggests that the absence of a spouse significantly increases the odds of coresidence with a child (Tsuya and Martin 1992; Tabuchi 1998; Yashiro 1999; Suzuki 2001; Tabuchi and Nakazato 2004). Thus, improvement to joint survivorship among elderly couples can contribute to a declining propensity to live with children. In fact, the percentage of currently married elderly women rose from 37.3 % in 1980 to 49.6 % in 2010. The literature also suggests that the odds of coresidence are significantly higher among agricultural households (Kojima 1989; Yashiro 1999) and lower in metropolitan areas (Tsuya and Martin 1992; Tabuchi 1998; Suzuki 2001; Tabuchi and Nakazato 2004). Thus, it is likely that industrialization and urbanization have also promoted this change. However, the most important cause could be the shift in social norms from stem families to nuclear families.

Although the percentage declined significantly, the propensity for the elderly to live with children is still higher in Japan than in Western developed countries. According to Iacovou (2000), the percentage living with children was less than 20 % in Northern/Protestant Europe and between 20 % and 40 % in Southern/Catholic Europe. This implies that the role of family as a "latent asset" in elderly-care is more important in Japan than in Europe.

6.2.2 Living Arrangements of the Elderly in Eastern Asia

Table 23 compares the living arrangements of the elderly people in four Eastern Asian countries, according to the 2010 census results. The propensity to live with children seems to be higher in the other Eastern Asian countries than in Japan.

Table 23 Living arrangements of elderly aged 65 and over in 2010 (%)

	Japan	Korea	Taiwan	China
Living alone	16.4	19.7	14.3	12.1
Couple only	33.7	77.7	19.6	11.4
Living with child	40.7		52.2	76.5
Other private households	3.5		11.3	
Institutional households	5.7	2.6	2.6	

Source 2010 census of each country

Although data on detailed living arrangements are not available in Korea's 2010 census, 55.0 % of the elderly heads of households comprising two or more persons coresided with children. Since a rough estimate for this figure in Japan based on family type is 22.5 %, it is likely that the percentage in Korea living with children is higher. Although estimation is difficult for China, it is possible that more than 70 % of elderly people there are living with children.

While the percentage living with children seems to be lowest in Japan, the propensity to live alone is highest in Korea. What is unique in Korea is the urban–rural divide. As shown in Table 24, living alone is the urban lifestyle for the elderly Japanese. On the other hand, the propensity to live alone is extremely high in rural areas of Korea, and the country's higher percentage compared to Japan is mainly due to their difference in rural areas. There was a major change in the administrative areas in Taiwan in 2010. However, the change does not affect the conclusion that there is practically no rural–urban difference there in terms of living alone. The difference is minimal in China as well.

The extremely high percentage of elderly living alone in rural Korea corresponds to the extremely advanced population aging. As shown in Table 25, rural populations tend to be older than urban populations in all countries, due to the rural–urban migration. However, the rural–urban difference in Korea is extremely large and suggests a level of rural–urban migration is much higher than in other countries. It is assumed that this large amount of rural–urban migration among members of younger generations has left behind elderly parents in rural areas and resulted in a high percentage of elderly individuals living alone.

On the other hand, the rural–urban difference in Taiwan is small even if the new administrative definition is applied. Considering the smaller land area than Korea and the similar level of economic development, the contrast between Korea and Taiwan is of special interest.

6.2.3 Urbanization in Korea and Taiwan

According to the 2010 census, the urban (i.e., city) population accounted for 82.0 % of Korea's total population. Taiwan's percentage of urban population in the 2010 census was 31.3 % according to the old definition and 65.7 % according to the new

Table 24 Proportion of elderly living alone by area in 2010 (%)

	Japan	Korea	Taiwan [a]	Taiwan [b]	China
Whole country	16.4	19.7	14.3	14.3	12.1
City	16.8	17.3	14.4	14.6	11.8
Town	13.1	21.5	14.2	14.2	12.5
Village		25.7			12.2

Source 2010 census of each country
[a] The former Taipei, Taichung, Tainan and Kaohsiung prefectures are included to cities
[b] The former Taipei, Taichung, Tainan and Kaohsiung prefectures are included to prefectures

Table 25 Proportion of elderly by area in 2010 (%)

	Japan	Korea	Taiwan [a]	Taiwan [b]	China
Whole Country	22.8	11.3	10.6	10.6	8.9
City	22.4	9.2	9.7	10.4	7.7
Town	26.7	13.5	12.3	10.7	8.0
Village		27.8			10.1

Source 2010 census of each country
[a] The former Taipei, Taichung, Tainan and Kaohsiung prefectures are included to cities
[b] The former Taipei, Taichung, Tainan and Kaohsiung prefectures are included to prefectures

definition. The change in regional distribution was also much more marked in Korea. The capital area of Korea consists of Seoul city, Incheon city, and Gyeonggi-do, accounting for 11.8 % of the whole land area. The share of national population within the capital area has rapidly increased, from 28.2 % in 1970 to 48.9 % in 2010. In Taiwan, there has been a cumulative concentration in the northern region that consists of Taipei city, New Taipei city (the former Taipei prefecture), Keelung city, Hsinchu city, Ilan prefecture, Taoyuan prefecture, and Hsinchu prefecture (Lin 2006). This region accounts for 20.4 % of Taiwan's land area. However, the share of population within this region increased from 34.3 % in 1970 to 46.3 % in 2010; the change was less drastic than that of Korea's capital area.

The contrast between the marked urbanization in Korea and the mild urbanization in Taiwan has its roots in colonial periods. Japan colonized Taiwan between 1895 and 1945, and Korea between 1910 and 1945. According to Chang Se-Hoon (2002), the accelerated industrialization in Korea during the colonial period produced a considerable amount of out-migration from the rural areas. However, the urbanization within the peninsula was curbed because many farmers had migrated abroad. However, return migration after 1945 and refugees from the north during the Korean War in 1950–1953 triggered extremely compressed urbanization. The process has been further exacerbated by economic development since the 1960s. Urbanization has become so marked that rural areas have been left underdeveloped and economic inequality between areas has rapidly grown.

Unlike in Korea where the rural economy was decimated, the agriculture sector in Taiwan in the early twentieth century was very competitive. While Korean farmers had nothing but rice to export, Taiwanese farmers exported sugar, camphor, tea, liquor, fruit, and straw hats. While the share of primary industry within GDP in Korea dropped from 58.4 % in 1920 to 43.1 % in 1940, in Taiwan within the same timeframe, it dropped only slightly from 37.8 to 36.0 % (Kim Nak-Nyeon 2004b). In the course of industrialization, land ownership in Korea and Japan became increasingly concentrated in the hands of large landlords. In Taiwan, however, land and wealth distribution became more equal in 1931–1945, thanks to the competitiveness of agricultural products (Cumings 1997). On account of this competitiveness, rural areas in Taiwan could accumulate capital and develop their infrastructure.

Since the mid-1960s, in Taiwan, light industry has grown mainly in the rural areas. Rural factories that produce textiles, plastic, and electric products absorbed the surplus population, thus precluding rapid urbanization (Ishida 2005). While Korean government sought to foster a small number of gigantic *jaebol*, a large number of small-sized companies in Taiwan grew through trade with the United States and Japan. The Taiwanese government protected these industries that were based in rural areas (Vogel 1991). Thus, Taiwan could avoid both drastic population aging and radical changes to the living arrangements of the elderly in rural areas.

6.3 Pension and Retirement

6.3.1 Pension Programs in Eastern Asia

Although occupational pensions for soldiers and government workers in Japan started in the nineteenth century, universal coverage in public pension and health insurance extending to all citizens was established in 1961. Japan's current system consists of three occupational pension plans; Employees' Pension (for workers in private companies), National Pension (for farmers and self-employed workers), and Mutual Aid Pension (for civil servants). Functionally, the current system contains three tiers. The first tier is the Basic Pension, which provides a flat rate of universal coverage. The second tier is the Employees' Pension Insurance, which is income-related in terms of both its premium and benefit structure. The third tier is an optional scheme. For the National Pension, the eligibility to receive pension benefits requires 25 years of premium payments. Major reforms were made in 2004, including the cutting back of future benefits, premium increases, and delaying the pensionable age from 60 to 65 years (NIPSSR 2011).

Early and occupation-specific pension programs in Korea included the Government Employees Pension, established in 1960; the Military Serviceman Pension, in 1963; and the Private School Teacher's Pension, in 1975. When the National Pension of Korea was established in 1988, it covered only employees at factories that employed 10 or more workers. The coverage expanded gradually to become universal in 1999 (Choi Sung-Jae 2000; Kim Yeong-Woo 2001). While Japan introduced a universal pension program in 1961 when the country's percentage of the elderly was 5.8 %, the figure for Korea was 6.8 % in 1999. Thus, Korea was slower than Japan in introducing a universal pension plan (Chang Byung-Won 2001a). The influence of Confucian familistic values is often referenced as one of reasons for this delay (Chang Kyung-Sup 2001; Kim Myoung-Jung 2004a; Kim Hyung-Nam 2010). Because having access to full benefits requires 20 years of contribution, the system will remain immature until 2019. Elderly people can receive 50–95 % of the full benefits if they contributed for 10–19 years, and 25–45 % if they contributed for 5–9 years. In 2009, 24.5 % of those who 65 and over received some benefit, but the amount was small because most of the recipients had contributed for fewer than 10 years (Kim Sung-Won 2011).

In Taiwan, the Kuomintang government planned in 2000 to introduce a universal pension plan. However, the Democratic Progressive Party (DPP) took power in 2000 and postponed the plan, choosing instead to prior recovery from the 9.21 earthquake in 1999, as well as economic development. It was in 2008 that a universal pension plan was finally introduced in Taiwan (Chen Hsiao-Hung 2009). This implies that elderly individuals living in Taiwan are largely supported by their families. According to the findings in the Senior Citizen Condition Survey in 2009 (Ministry of the Interior 2009), the importance of children and children-in-law for economic support (49.29 %) was ranked the highest, followed by public welfare (29.66 %), retirement money and pension (17.37 %), and own income (14.93 %).

In 1951, China introduced a socialist pension system that did not require premium payments. In the wake of economic reforms since the 1980s, however, this socialist system has covered only government workers. A pension program for private company workers and the self-employed in urban areas was established in 1997. It was in 2009 that rural residents of China were finally covered by a pension program. According to the 2010 census, while 66.3 % of the urban elderly in China relied on pension benefits, only 4.6 % of the rural elderly received it (Ling Li et al. 2011). The Chinese government relies on families to provide support to the elderly, and this reliance is more obvious in China than in other Eastern Asian countries. The Law on Protection of the Rights and Interests of the Elderly, enacted in 1996, allows elderly parents to demand financial support from their children. A 2013 revision made it obligatory for children to visit their elderly parents frequently.

6.3.2 Labor Force Participation Among Elderly Males

Figure 38 compares the rate of male labor force participation among Eastern Asian countries in 2010. In Japan, the rate is sustained until ages 55–59 and suddenly starts to decline after age 60. This suggests that most Japanese male workers remain at the work-place until the official retirement age of 60. On the other hand,

Fig. 38 Male labor force participation rates in 2010

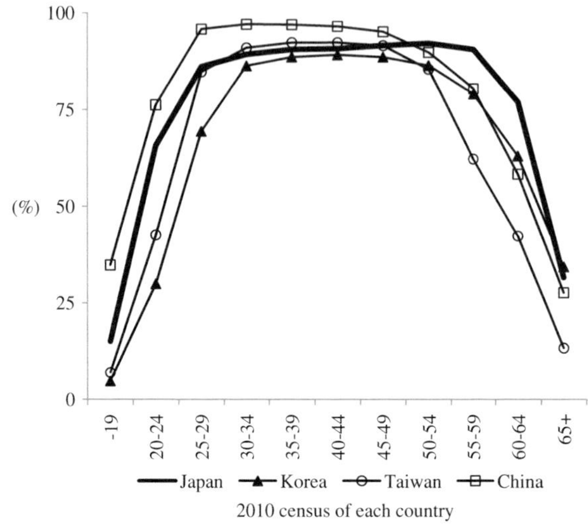

the rates in other Eastern Asian countries start to decline in the fifties. This suggests that the lifetime employment is not as prevalent in those countries as in Japan, and that older workers find it difficult to secure employment once they are pushed out of the work-place.

According to An Chong-Bum, et al. (2011), older workers in Korea suffer from a disadvantage, given the country's rapid changes in technological progress and education attainment. According to newspapers, the age discrimination against older workers is expressed in such Korean phrases as "*sa-o-jeong*" ("retiring at age 45 is usual") or "*o-ryuk-tu*" ("staying until age 56 makes one a thief"). It is likely that older workers in Taiwan and China are experiencing the same problem. In addition to slow developments of social security (including pension), lower rates of labor force participation make the role of familial support more important in those countries than in Japan.

6.4 Politics of Population Aging

As the most aged country in the world, Japan's public expenditure toward the elderly has been so large that adjustments are often required. In addition to the 2004 pension reforms, a new medical insurance system for those aged 75 and over was established in 2008. The consumption tax rate will be raised from the current 5 to 8 % in 2014 and 10 % in 2015. From that money, at most JPY 0.6 trillion is earmarked to improve the pension program; at most JPY 1.6 trillion to extend medical care and long-term care programs; and JPY 0.7 trillion to fund pro-natal interventions. Naturally, such resource allocations have political implications; and radical or ambitious proposals may not surface for a sometime, following the DPJ's failure to keep its election promise.

It is likely that elderly Koreans are in more serious conditions than the Japanese, given their country's slower development of a security net and more drastic changes in the living arrangements. Because a radical transformation is required in this area, political leaders tend to make ambitious proposals. President Park Geun-Hye apologized in September 2013 for the failure to keep promises made during the election; such failure can result in low trust with regard to policy-makers and harm the effectiveness of interventions.

Taiwanese elderly seem to be better protected by the family than their Korean counterparts. As suggested in Table 10, traditional Confucian values are most robust in Taiwan. Change in living arrangements among the elderly was less pronounced there, due to the less drastic urbanization. In the 2012 presidential election campaign, neither of the main parties discussed the welfare of the elderly, but worried the low income and poverty of younger generations. Furthermore, the relationship with mainland China is so overwhelming that other political issues tend to attract relatively little interest.

Unlike the governments of advanced democratic countries, the Chinese government explicitly attempts to enforce familial support for elderly parents. The 1980 constitution defined that both parents and children have obligations with regard to mutual support. The Marriage Law in 1980 stated that a parent can demand monetary support from a child who does not fulfill this obligation (Yuyama 2006). The aforementioned Law on Protection of the Rights and Interests of the Elderly further emphasizes filial-piety obligations. The traditional Confucian values in China, it seems, were destroyed systematically during the Cultural Revolution. It appears to be difficult for the government to induce the restoration of old values.

6.5 Conclusion

While Japan is presently the most aged country in the world, it is likely that Eastern Asia will become the most aged region. Since the development of social security system has been slow in Eastern Asia, the need for familial support of the elderly will likely escalate as the population ages. This can discourage individuals from having children and thus create a vicious circle of fertility decline and population aging.

According to Lee (2007), the impact of a "second dividend" of population aging on economic growth depends on the sources of income among the elderly. However, the shares of asset-based reallocation in Japan and Taiwan are smaller than in the United States and Thailand, for example. This implies that population aging could depress the Eastern Asian economy more seriously than the economies of other regions.

7 Concluding Remarks

Japan was the first non-European developed country and was the only exception for a long time in the Eurocentric developed world. However, Asian newly industrialized economies including Korea and Taiwan succeeded in economic take-off after the 1970s, and they have been followed by China since the 1990s. Thus, economic development and high living standards are no longer limited to the offshoots of European civilization. It has turned out, however, that the discrepancy between the rapidly changing socioeconomic systems and the slower-to-change family systems is greater in Eastern Asia than in Europe or Anglo-Saxon countries. Because industrialization and post-industrialization were led by Anglo-Saxon countries, Northern/Western European families are thought to be most adaptive and advantageous. On the other hand, Eastern Asian families, especially Confucian families, have difficulty to adjust to the postindustrial system. Such maladjustment has supposedly resulted in extremely low fertility and drastic population aging.

Japan's demographic bonus ended in the 1990s, and the total dependency ratio started to increase and the working-age population started to decline. It is difficult to evaluate the degree to which such a demographic background affected Japan's economic recession after the 1990s. However, it is obvious that the declining labor supply should depress the economic growth. In addition, it is unlikely that population aging in Eastern Asia boost economic growth through the second dividend, as asset-based reallocation by the elderly there is uncommon. Thus, economic growth in the non-European world is likely to be obstructed by population aging at earlier stages than those seen with the European forerunners.

Because Latin American countries are offshoots of European civilization, fertility decline there following their economic take-off could resemble the scenario seen in Southern Europe. However, if the economies of India or the Islamic countries were to arrive at the level of Eastern Asia in 2000, the misalignment with the family system could be even larger than that currently seen in Eastern Asia. In such cases, fertility could drop like a proverbial stone, population aging could become even more drastic, and economic growth could be checked at an even earlier stage. Such a mechanism could contribute to the sustenance of the Eurocentric system, as asserted in dependency theory or world-system theory.

Although the Japanese economy has actually slowed, the full impact of population aging on the rapidly growing Eastern Asian economy has not yet been determined. It is possible that some cultural features could improve labor productivity or promote innovation, and thus compensate for negative demographic impacts. It is also possible that the family system will quickly adjust to the postindustrial setting, and that fertility will recover more quickly than predicted. We need to continue to make observations, if we are to know whether the Eastern Asian economy is actually being checked by the predicted rapid population aging.

Japan became one of the major role players in the early 20th century, and challenged liberal democracy as a member of the axis of totalism. Following its defeat in World War II, Japan shifted to a liberal democracy and developed the second-largest economy in the world. Although Korea and Taiwan have succeeded in terms of economic growth under developmental dictatorships, the two countries also became liberal democracies in the late 1980s. On the other hand, China recently surpassed Japan to become the second-largest economy worldwide, while sustaining the odd amalgamation of a socialist dictatorship and a market economy. Whether or not the Chinese economy is checked by early aging has special importance in human history, for it will determine the sustainability of the Eurocentric world system and the validity of the conclusion asserted by Fukuyama (1992) that the Western liberal democracy is the ultimate form of human government.

References

An, Chong-Bum, Chun Young-Jun, Gim Eul-Sik, Hwang Namhui, and Lee Sang-Hyop. 2011. Integenerational resource allocation in the republic of Korea. In *Population Aging and the Generational Economy*, ed. Ronald Lee, and Andrew Mason, 381–393. Cheltenham: Edward Elgar.

Arita, Shin. 2006. *Kankoku-no Kyoiku to Shakai Kaiso: 'Gakureki Shakai' -heno Jisshoteki Approach* (*Education and Social Stratification in South Korea: An Empirical Approach to the 'School Credential Society'*) (in Japanese). Tokyo: University of Tokyo Press.

Asami, Yasushi, Koichi Ishizaka, Moriyuki Oe, Yasuyo Koyama, Sachiko Segawa, and Masumi Matsumoto. 2000. Shoshika gensho to jutaku jijo (Low fertility phenomena and housing conditions) (in Japanese). *Jinko Mondai Kenkyu (Journal of Population Problems)* 56(1): 8–37.

Atoh, Makoto. 1992. Nihon-ni okeru shusseiritsu-no doko to yoin (in Japanese). In *Teishussei-wo Meguru Shomondai*, eds. Kono Shigemi, and Minoru Okada, 48–68. Tokyo: Daimindo.

Atoh, Makoto. 2000. *Gendai Jinkogaku: Shoshi Koreika-no Kiso Chisiki* (in Japanese). Tokyo: Nihon Hyoronsha.

Atoh, Makoto, and Akachi Mayuko. 2003. Nhon-no shoshika to kazoku seisaku: Kokusai hikaku-no kanten-kara (Below-replacement fertility and family policy in Japan in an international comparative perspective) (in Japanese). *Jinko Mondai Kenkyu (Journal of Population Problems)* 59(1): 27–48.

Becker, Gary S. 1991. *A Treatise on the Family, Enlarged Edition*. Cambridge: Harvard University Press.

Billari, Francesco C. 2008. Lowest-low fertility in Europe: Exploring the causes and finding some surprises. *The Japanese Journal of Population* 6(1): 1–18.

Billari, Francesco, Dimiter Philipov, and Pau Baizán. 2001. Leaving home in Europe: The experience of cohorts born around 1960. Max Planck Institute for Demographic Research, WP2001-014.

Billari, Francesco C., and Hans-Peter Kohler. 2002. Patterns of lowest-low fertility in Europe. Max Planck Institute for Demographic Research Working Paper WP-2002-040.

Boling, Patricia. 2007. Policies to support working mothers and children in Japan. In *Political Economy of Japan's Low Fertility*, ed. Frances McCall Rosenbluth, 131–154. Stanford: Stanford University Press.

Bongaarts, John. 1978. A framework for analyzing the proximate determinants of fertility. *Population and Development Review* 4(1): 105–132.

Bongaarts, John, and Griffith Feeney. 1998. On the quantum and tempo of fertility. *Population and Development Review* 24(2): 271–291.

Caldwell, John C. 2006. *Demographic Transition Theory*. Dordrecht: Springer.

Cha, Kyung-Wuk. 2005. Jeochulsan gagye-wa chulsan gyehoek issneun gagye-eui gyeongje gujo bigyo bunseok (The difference in household economic structure between low-fertility and birth-planned households) (in Korean). *Hanguk Gajeong Gwanri Hakhoeji (Journal of Korean Home Management Association)* 23(2): 137–148.

Chang, Byung-Won. 2001a. Shakaihosho, shakaifukushi-ni okeru nikkan hikaku: Koreika shakai shoki dankai-no shojokyo to seisaku doko-wo chushin-ni (in Japanese). *Kaigai Shakai Hosho Kenkyu (The Review of Comparative Social Security Research)* 135: 81–97.

Chang, Kyung-Sup. 2001b. Abchukjeok geundaeseong-gwa noinmunje-eui jaeinsik: 'Shinsede' roseoeui noin (Compressed modernity and reconception of the aging issue: Aged people as 'new generation') (in Korean). *Kajok-gwa Munhwa (Journal of the Korean Family Studies Association)* 13(1): 1–29.

Chang, Kyung-Sup. 2002a. Hanguk gajok-eui 'jeongsang wigi'? Ubaljeok daweonseong-gwa gineungjok gwabuka-reul jungshim-euro (The 'normal crisis' of Korean families? Focusing on accidental pluralism and functional overloading) (in Korean). *Hanguk-eui Yeseol (Korean Decorum)* 4: 11–35.

Chang, Ming-Cheng. 2003. Demographic transition in Taiwan. *Journal of Population and Social Security: Population Study* 1: 611–628.

Chang, Se-Hoon. 2002. Doshihwa (in Korean). In *Hanguk-eui Ingu*, eds. Doo-Sub Kim, Sang-Tae Park, and Ki-Soo Eun, 495–523. National Statistics Office.

Chang, Kyung-Sup, et al. 2006. *Gyeongje, Sahoejeok Yanggeukhwa Shidae-eui Gajokjeongchaek* (in Korean). Ministry of Gender Equality and Family, Yeongu Bogo 2006–2013.

Chen, Hsiao-Hung. 2009. Taiwan shakai seisaku-no hatten: shisa to Tenbo (in Japanese). In *Higashi Asia-no Shakai Hosho: Nihon, Kankoku, Taiwan-no Genjo to Kadai*, eds. Takafumi Uzubashi, Kiyomi Kimura, and Hiroyuki Totani, 138–163. Kyoto: Nakanishiya Shuppan.

Choi, Sung-Jae. 2000. Aging in Korea. In *Ageing in the Asia-Pacific Region*, ed. David R. Phillips, 223–242. London: Routledge.

Choi, Eun-Young. 2008. Kankoku-no aratana shakaiteki risk: Shigoto to katei-no ryoritsu, shotoku kakusa (New social risks in Korea: Balancing work and family, income polarization) (in Japanese). *Kaigai Shakai Hosho Kenkyu (The Review of Comparative Social Security Research)* 163: 65–79.

Choi, Eun-Young, et al. 2005. *Hanguk-eui Jeochulsan Gwanyeon Sahoe Gyeongjejeok Yoin-gwa Jeongchaek Yeogeon* (in Korean). Korea Institute for Health and Social Affairs, Gyeongje Inmun Sahoe Yeongguhoe Habdong Yeongu Chongso 05-14-2002.

Chu, C. Y. Cyrus, and Ruoh-Rong Yu. 2010. *Understanding Chinese Families: A Comparative study of Taiwan and Southeast China*. Oxford: Oxford University Press.

Council for Economic Planning and Development, Executive Yuan (Xingzehngyuan JingJi Jianshe Weiyuanhui). 2010. *2010-nian zhi 2060-nian Taiwan Renkou Tuiji* (in Chinese).

Cumings, Bruce. 1997. Japanese colonialism in Korea: A comparative perspective. http://aparc.stanford.edu/publications/japanese_colonialism_in_korea_a_comparative_perspective/ Accessed 19 November 2013.

Cumings, Bruce. 2005. Korea's Place in the Sun: A Modern History, Updated Edition. New York: W. W. Norton & Co.

d'Addio, Anna Cristina, and Marco Mira d'Ercole. 2005. Trends and determinants of fertility rates in OECD countries: The role of policies. *CECD Social, Employment and Migration Working Papers* 27.

Dalla Zuanna, Gianpiero. 2001. The banquet of Aeolus: A familistic interpretation of Italy's lowest low fertility. *Demographic Research* 4(5): 1–21.

Directorate-General of Budget, Accounting and Statistics, Executive Yuan (Xingzhengyuan Zhuji Zongsuo). 2003. *Funu Honyu yu Jiuye Diaocha (Report on Fertility and Employment of Married Women)* (in Chinese).

Directorate-General of Budget, Accounting and Statistics, Executive Yuan (Xingzhengyuan Zhuji Zongsuo). 2013. Woguo HDI, GII fenbie paiming quanqiu di 23-wei ji di 2-wei (in Chinese). *Guoqing Tongji Tongbao* No. 105.

Easterlin, R.A. 1978. What will 1984 be like? Socioeconomic implications of recent twists in age structure. *Demography* 15(4): 397–421.

Eisenstadt, S. N. 1996. *Japanese Civilization: A Comparative View*. Chicago: University of Chicago Press.

Engelhardt, Henriette and Alexia Prskawetz. 2005. A pooled time-series analysis on the relation between fertility and female employment. IUSSP XXV International Population Conference, Tours.

Eun, Ki-Soo. 2003. Understanding recent fertility decline in Korea. *Journal of Population and Social Security: Population Study* 1: 574–595.

Eun, Ki-Soo. 2005. Mihon-eseo gyeolhon-euro ihaeng: Choegeun urinara-eseo jeochulsan-e gachneun euimi. (Transition from single to marriage) (in Korean). *Bogon Bokchi Forum* 102: 25–35.

Feeney, Griffith, and Andrew Mason. 2001. Population in East Asia. In *Population Changes and Economic Development in East Asia,* ed. Andrew Mason, 61–95. Stanford: Stanford University Press.

Frejka, Tomas, and Gérald Calot. 2001. Cohort reproductive patterns in low-fertility countries. *Population and Development Review* 27(1): 103–132.

Fujino, Atsuko. 2002. Kakei-ni okeru shussei kodo to tsuma-no shugyo kodo: Otto-no kaji ikuji sanka to tsuma-no kachikan-no eikyo (Fertility behavior and labor supply of married women in Japan: The impact of a husband's participation in household work and a wife's family values) (in Japanese). *Jinkogaku Kenkyu (The Journal of Population Studies)* 31: 19–35.

Fukuyama, Francis. 1992. *The End of History and the Last Man*. New York: Free Press.

Fukuyama, Francis. 1995. *Trust: The Social Virtues and the Creation of Prosperity*. New York: Free Press.

Gauthier, Anne H. 2002. Family policies in industrialized countries: Is there convergence ? *Population (English Edition)* 57(3): 447–474.

Goldscheider, Francis K., and Calvin Goldscheider. 1994. Leaving and returning home in 20th century America. *Population Bulletin* 48(4): 1–35.

Goldstein, Joshua R., Tomas Sobotka, and Aiva Jasilioniene. 2009. The end of 'lowest-low' fertility? *Population and Development Review* 35(4): 663–699.

Goode, William J. 1963. *World Revolution and Family Patterns*. New York: The Free Press of Glencoe.

Griffis, William Elliot. 1876. *The Mikado's Empire*. New York: Harper.

Gu, Baochang. 2009. The arrival of low fertility in China. In *Ultra-low Fertility in Pacific Asia,* eds. Gavin Jones, P. T. Straughan and Angelique Chan, 73–95. London: Routledge.

Hajnal, J. 1965. European marriage patterns in perspective, In *Population in History,* eds. D. V. Glass, and D. E. C. Eversley, 101–143. Chicago: Aldine Publishing.

Hajnal, J. 1982. Two kinds of preindustrial household formation system. *Population and Development Review* 8(3): 449–494.

Halman, Loek, Ronald Inglehart, Jaime Díez-Medrano, Ruud Juijkx, Alejandro Moreno, and Miguel Basáñez. 2008. *Changing Values and Beliefs in 85 Countries: Trends from the Values Surveys from 1981 to 2004*. Leiden: Koninklijke Brill.

Hardee-Cleaveland, Karen, and Judith Bannister. 1988. Fertility policy and implementation in China. *Population and Development Review* 14(2): 245–286.

Haruki, Ikumi. 2006. *Gendai Kankoku to Josei* (in Japanese). Tokyo: Sinkansha.

Hayashi, Yoshikoto. 1997. *Chugoku Kindai Seiji to Jukyo Bunka* (in Japanese). Tokyo: Toho Shoten.

Hirosima, Kiyosi. 1983. Sengo nihon-ni okeru oya to ko-no dokyoritsu-no keishiki jinkogakuteki bunseki model (Formal demography of parent-child coresidentiality in postwar Japan) (in Japanese). *Jinko Mondai Kenkyu (Journal of Population Problems)* 167: 18–31.

Hirosima, Kiyosi. 1984. Sengo nihon-ni okeru oya to ko-no dokyoritsu-no jinkogakuteki jissho bunseki (Demographic analysis of parent-child co-residentiality in postwar Japan) (in Japanese). *Jinko Mondai Kenkyu (Journal of Population Problems)* 169: 31–42.

Hirosima, Kiyosi. 2000. Kinnen-no gokei shusseiritsu teika-no yoin bunkai: Fufu shusseiritsu-wa teikashiteinaika? (Decomposition of the decline in the total fertility rate since 1970s in Japan: Has not married fertility affected?) (in Japanese). *Jinkogaku Kenkyu (The Journal of Population Studies)* 26: 1–20.

Hirosima, Kiyosi. 2001. Shusseiritsu teika-wo donoyoni toraeruka? Nenreibetsu yuhaigu shusseiritsu-no mondaisei (How to analyze fertility deceline?: Drawback in age-specific marital fertility rate) (in Japanese). *Riron to Hoho (Sociological Theory and Methods)* 16(2): 163–183.

Hirosima, Kiyosi. 1999. Kekkon to shussei-no shakai jinkogaku (in Japanese). *In Koza Shakaigaku 2: Kazoku (Sociology in Japan 2: Family Sociology)*, eds. Yoriko Meguro, and Hideki Watanabe, 21–57. Tokyo: University of Tokyo Press.

Hoem, Jan M., Alexia Prskawetz, and Gerda Neyer. 2001. Autonomy or conservative adjustment? The effect of public policies and educational attainment on third births in Austria, 1975–1996. *Population Studies* 55(3): 249–261.

Hoorens, Stijin, Andrew Parkinson, and Jonathan Grant. 2005. Sweden's varying success in offsetting low fertility. International Conference on Low Fertility and Effectiveness of Policy Measures in OECD, Seoul, Korea.

Hoshi, Atsuhi. 2007. Support network-ga shussei kodo to ishiki-ni ataeru eikyo (Effects of the support networks on fertility behaviors and attitudes) (in Japanese). *Jinko Mondai Kenkyu (Journal of Population Problems)* 63(4): 14–27.

Huntington, Samuel P. 1996. *The Clash of Civilizations and the Remaking of World Order*. New York: Free Press.

Iacovou, Maria. 2000. The living arrangements of elderly Europeans. ISER working paper 2000–2009.

Inglehart, Ronald, and Pippa Norris. 2003. *Rising Tide: Gender Equality and Cultural Change around the World*. Cambridge: Cambridge University Press.

Inglehart, Ronald, and Christian Welzel. 2008. *Modernization, Cultural Change, and Democracy: The Human Development Sequence*. Cambridge: Cambridge University Press.

Institute of Population Problems (Koseisho Jinko Mondai Kenkyuujo). 1982. *Nihon-no Shorai Suikei Jinko: Showa 56-nen 11-gatsu Suikei (Future Population Projections for Japan: Prepared in November 1981)* (in Japanese). Research Series No. 227.

Institute of Population Problems (Koseisho Jinko Mondai Kenkyuujo). 1987. *Nihon-no Shorai Suikei Jinko: Showa 61-nen 12-gatsu Suikei (Population projections for Japan: 1985-2085)* (in Japanese). Research Series No. 244.

Institute of Population Problems (Koseisho Jinko Mondai Kenkyuujo). 1992. *Nihon-no Shorai Suikei Jinko: Heisei 4-nen 9-gatsu Suikei (Population projections for Japan: 1991-2090)* (in Japanese). Research Series No. 274.

Ishida, Hiroshi. 2005. *Taiwan Minshuka to Chutai Keizai Kankei: Seiji-no Naikoka to Keizai-no Gaikoka* (*Studies of Taiwan's Democratization and Its Economic Relationship with China*) (in Japanese). Osaka: Kansai University Press.

Iwai, Noriko, and Yasuda Tokio. 2009. *Data-de Miru Higashi Asia-no Kazokukan: Higashi Asia Shakai Chosa-ni yoru Nikkanchutai no Hikaku* (in Japanese). Kyoto: Nakanishiya Shuppan.

Iwasawa, Miho. 2002. Kinnen-no TFR hendo-ni okeru kekkon kodo oyobi fufu-no shussei kodo-no henka-no kiyo-ni tsuite (On the contribution of the changes in first marriage behavior and couple's reproductive behavior to the recent change in total fertility rates of Japan) (in Japanese). *Jinko Mondai Kenkyu (Journal of Population Problems)* 58(3): 15–44.

Jun, Kwang-Hee. 2003. Hanguk-eui chulsanryeok byeoncheon: Chui-wa yeocheuk (Fertility transition in Korea: Trend and prospect) (in Korean). *Tongye Yeongu* 8(1): 35–58.

Kaneko, Ryuichi. 2004. Shoshika-no jinkogakuteki mechanism (in Japanese). In *Shoshika-no Jinkogaku*. eds. Hiroshi Obuchi, and Shigesato Takahashi, 15–36. Tokyo: Hara Shobo.

Kawashima, Takeyoshi. 1957. *Ideology-toshiteno Kazoku Seido* (in Japanese). Tokyo: Iwanami Shoten.

Kim, Yeong-Woo. 2001. Kankoku-ni okeru koteki nenkin seido-no doko (Recent trends in public pensions of Korea) (in Japanese). *Kaigai Shakai Hosho Kenkyu (The Review of Comparative Social Security Research)* 137: 86–94.

Kim, Myoung-Jung. 2004a. IMF taisei iko-no kankoku-no shakai keizai-no henka to koteki, shiteki shakai sishutu-no doko (The trend of public and private social expenditure and recent changes in the social economy after the introduction of the IMF program in Korea) (in Japanese). *Kaigai Shakai Hosho Kenkyu (The Review of Comparative Social Security Research)* 146: 4–22.

Kim, Seung-Kwon. 2004b. Choegeun hanguk sahoe-eui chulsanyul byeonhwa-eui weonin-gwa hyanghu jeonmang (Canges in fertility rates in Korea: Causes and future prospects) (in Korean). *Hanguk Inguhak (Korea Journal of Population Studies)* 27(2): 1–33.

Kim, Doo-Sub. 2005. Theoretical explanations of rapid fertility decline in Korea. *The Japanese Journal of Population* 3: 2–25.

Kim, Sung-Won. 2011. Kankoku-ni okeru nenkin seido to josei: Kohatsukoku-no bunmyaku-kara (Women and the pension system in South Korea: In the context of the late-coming welfare state) (in Japanese). *Kaigai Shakai Hosho Kenkyu (The Review of Comparative Social Security Research)* 175: 70–82.

Kim, Il-Gon. 1992. *Higashi Asia-no Keizai Hatten to Jukyo Bunka* (in Japanese). Tokyo: Daishukan Shoten.

Kim, Nak-Nyeon. 2004. Shokuminchiki Taiwan to Chosen-no kogyoka (in Japanese). In *Nihon Shihonshugi to Chosen, Taiwan: Teikokushugika-no Keizai Hendo (Modern Japanese Capitalism and Korea and Taiwan: Structural Change under Japan's Imperial Rule)*, eds. Kazuo Hori, and Satoshi Nakamura, 135–162. Kyoto: Kyoto University Press.

Kim, Hyung-Nam. 2010. Kankoku-no koreisha mondai to koreisha fukushi seisaku (in Japanese). In *Gendai Kankoku-no Kazoku Seisaku*, eds. Kimio Ito, Ikumi Haruki, and Hyung-Nam Kim, 121–138. Kyoto: Korosha.

Kohler, Hans-Peter, Francesco C. Billari, and José Antonio Ortega. 2002. The emergence of lowest-low fertility in Europe during the 1990s. *Population and Development Review* 28(4): 641–681.

Kojima, Hiroshi. 1989. Intergenerational household extension in Japan. In *Ethnicity and the New Family Economy*, ed. Frances K. Goldscheider, and Calvin Goldscheider, 163–184. Boulder, Colorado: Westview Press.

Kono, Shigemi. 1995. Haigu kankei to shusseiryoku (in Japanese). In *Gendai Nihon-no Jinko Mondai*, ed. Nihon Tokei Kyokai, 63–110. Tokyo: Okurasho Insatsukyoku.

Lee, Ronald D. 1994. The formal demography of population aging, transfers, and the economic life cycle. In *Demography of Aging*, ed. Linda G. Martin, and Samuel H. Preston, 8–49. Washington DC: National Academy Press.

Lee, Ronald D. 2007. *Global Population Aging and its Economic Consequences*. Washington DC: AEI Press.

Lee, Meilin. 2009. Transition to below replacement fertility and policy response in Taiwan. *The Japanese Journal of Population* 7: 71–86.

Lee, Sam-Sik. 2009. Low fertility and policy responses in Korea. *The Japanese Journal of Population* 7: 57–70.

Lee, Sam-Sik, et al. 2005. *2005-nyeondo Jeonguk Gyeolhon mich Chulsan Dohyang Josa (2005 National Survey on Dynamics of Marriage and Fertility)* (in Korean). Korea Institute for Health and Social Affairs, Yeongu Bogoso 2005–30(1).

Lee, Sam-Sik, et al. 2009. *2009-nyeondo Jeonguk Gyeolhon mich Chulsan Dohyang Josa* (*2009 National Survey on Dynamics of Marriage and Fertility)* (in Korean). Korea Institute for Health and Social Affairs, Jeongchek Bogoso 2009–83.

Lesthaeghe, Ron. 2010. The unfolding story of the second demographic transition. *Population and Development Review* 36(2): 211–251.

Li, Ling, Chen Qiulin, and Yu. Jiang. 2011. The changing patterns of China's public services. In *Population Aging and the Generational Economy*, ed. Ronald Lee, and Andrew Mason, 408–420. Cheltenham: Edward Elgar.

Lin, Ji-Ping. 2006. The dynamics of labor migration in Taiwan: Evidence from the 1990 and 2000 Taiwan Population Censuses. *Geography Research Forum* 26: 61–92.
Livi-Bacci, M. 2001. Too few children and too much family. *Daedalus* 130(3): 139–156.
Lutz, W., V. Skirbekk, and M. R. Testa. 2006. The low fertility trap hypothesis: Forces that may lead to further postponement and fewer births in Europe. *Vienna Yearbook of Population Research 2006*, 115–151.
Mason, Andrew. 2001. Population and economic growth in East Asia In *Population Changes and Economic Development in East Asia,* ed. Andrew Mason, 1–30. Stanford: Stanford University Press.
Mason, Andrew, and Ronald Lee. 2012. Population aging and the generational economy: key findings. In *Population Aging and the Generational Economy*, ed. Ronald Lee, and Andrew Mason, 3–31. Cheltenham: Edward Elgar.
McDonald, Peter. 2000. Gender equity in theories of fertility transition. *Population and Development Review* 26(3): 427–440.
McDonald, Peter. 2002. Sustaining fertility through public policy: The range of options. *Population (English Edition)* 57(3): 417–446.
McDonald, Peter. 2008. Very low fertility: Consequences, causes and policy approaches. *The Journal of Japanese Population* 6(1): 19–23.
McDonald, Peter. 2005. Fertility and the state: The efficacy of policy. XXV International Population Conference.
McDonald, Peter. 2009. Explanations of low fertility in East Asia: A comparative perspective. In *Ultra-low fertility in Pacific Asia,* eds. Gavin Jones, P. T. Straughan, and Angelique Chan, 23–39. London: Routledge.
Meguro, Yoriko, and Hachiro Nishioka. 2000. Shoshika mondai-no gender bunseki (Gender analysis on fertility decline in Japan) (in Japanese). *Jinko Mondai Kenkyu (Journal of Population Problems)* 56(4): 38–69.
Micheli, Giuseppe A. 2000. Kinship, family and social network: The anthropological embedment of fertility change in Southern Europe. *Demographic Research* 3(13): 1–27.
Ministry of the Interior (Neizhengbu). 2009. *Zhonghua Minguo 98-nian Laoren Zhuangkuang Diaocha Baoguo (Report of the Senior Citizen Condition Survey 2009, Republic of China)* (in Chinese).
Ministry of the Interior (Neizhengbu). 2011. *Renkou Zhengce Bainian Huigu yu Zhanwang (Centenary Population Policy and Vision)* (in Chinese).
Morita, Yoko. 2006. Kosodate-ni tomonau disincentive-no kanwasaku (in Japanese). In *Shoshika to Nihon-no Keizai Shakai: Futatsu-no Shinwa to Hitotsu-no Shinjitsu*, ed. Yoshio Higuchi, 49–80. Tokyo: Nihon Hyoronsha.
Murphey, Rhoads. 2009. *East Asia: A New History, Fifth Edition.* New Jersey: Longman.
Naikakufu (Cabinet Office). 2005. *Heisei 17-nendo Shoshika-ni Kansuru Kokusai Hikaku Chosa* (in Japanese).
Nakane, Chie. 1970. *Kazoku-no Kozo: Shakai Jinruigakuteki Bunseki* (in Japanese). Tokyo: University of Tokyo Press.
National Institute of Population and Social Security Research. 2011. *Social Security in Japan 2011.*
National Institute of Population and Social Security Research (Kokuritsu Shakai Hosho Jinko Mondai Kenkyujo). 1997. *Nihon-no Shorai Suikei Jinko: Heisei 9-nen 1-gatsu Suikei (Population Projections for Japan: 1996–2100)* (in Japanese). Research Series No. 291.
National Institute of Population and Social Security Research (Kokuritsu Shakai Hosho Jinko Mondai Kenkyujo). 2002. *Nihon-no Shorai Suikei Jinko: Heisei 14-nen 1-gatsu Suikei (Population Projections for Japan: 2001–2050)* (in Japanese). Research Series No. 303.
National Institute of Population and Social Security Research (Kokuritsu Shakai Hosho Jinko Mondai Kenkyujo). 2007. *Nihon-no Shorai Suikei Jinko: Heisei 18-nen 12-gatsu Suikei (Population Projections for Japan: 2006–2055)* (in Japanese). Research Series No. 315.

National Institute of Population and Social Security Research (Kokuritsu Shakai Hosho Jinko Mondai Kenkyujo). 2012a. *Nihon-no Shorai Suikei Jinko: Heisei 24-nen 1-gatsu Suikei (Population Projections for Japan: 2011–2060)* (in Japanese). Research Series No. 326.

National Institute of Population and Social Security Research (Kokuritsu Shakai Hosho Jinko Mondai Kenkyujo). 2012b. *Dai 14-kai Shussho Doko Kihon Chosa dai-1 Hokokusho: Wagakuni Fufu-no Kekkon Katei to Shusshoryoku (Report on the Fourteenth Japanese National Fertility Survey in 2010: Marriage Process and Fertility of Japanese Married Couples)* (in Japanese). Survey Series No. 29.

National Institute of Population and Social Security Research (Kokuritsu Shakai Hosho Jinko Mondai Kenkyujo). 2013. *Jinko Tokei Siryoshu (Latest Demographic Statistics 2013)* (in Japanese). Population Research Series No. 328.

National Statistics Office (Tonggyecheong). 2009. *Tongye-ro Boneun Yeoseong-eui Sarm 2009* (in Korean).

National Statistics Office (Tonggyecheong). 2011. *Jangrae Ingu Chugye: 2010-nyeon–2060-nyeon* (in Korean).

National Statistics Office (Tonggyecheong). 2012. *Hanguk-eui Sahoe Jipyo 2012* (in Korean).

Ogawa, Naohiro. 2003. Japan's changing fertility mechanisms and its policy response. *Journal of Population Research* 20(1): 89–106.

Oi, Masako. 2004. Bubble hokai zengo-no shussan kosodate-no sedaikan sai (in Japanese). In *Joseitachi-no Heisei Fukyo: Defure-de Hatarakikata, Kurashi-wa Do Kawattaka*, eds. Higuchi Yoshio, Ota Kiyoshi, and Kakei Keizai Kenkyujo, 117–151. Tokyo: Nikkei Inc.

Oyama, Masako. 2004. Kodomo-no yoiku, kyoiku hiyo to shusseiritsu teika (Cost of raising children and the recent fertility decline in Japan) (in Japanese). *Jinkogaku Kenkyu (The Journal of Population Studies)* 35: 45–57.

Perry, Matthew Calbraith. 1856. *Narrative of the Expedition of an American Squadron to the China Seas and Japan*. Washington: A.O.P. Nicholson.

Population Problems Research Council, the Mainichi Newspapers (Mainichi Shinbunsha Jinko Mondai Chosakai). 2005. *Choshoshika Jidai-no Kazoku Ishiki: Dai 1-kai Jinko, Kazoku, Sedai Yoron Chosa Hokokusho* (in Japanese). Mainichi Newspapers.

Ravanera, Z.R., F. Rajulton, and T.K. Burch. 1995. A cohort analysis of home-leaving in Canada, 1910–1975. *Journal of Comparative Family Studies* 26(2): 179–193.

Reher, David Sven. 1998. Family ties in Western Europe: Persistent contrasts. *Population and Development Review* 24(2): 203–234.

Retherford, Robert D., and Naohiro Ogawa. 2006. Japan's baby bust: Casuses, implications, and policy responses. In *The Baby Bust: Who Will Do the Work? Who Will Pay the Taxes?* ed. Fred R. Harris, 5–47. Lanham, Maryland: Rowman and Littlefied.

Rosenbluth, Frances McCall. 2007. The political economy of low fertility. In *Political Economy of Japan's Low Fertility*, ed. Frances McCall Rosenbluth, 3–36. Stanford: Stanford University Press.

Sasai, Tsukasa. 1998. Kinnen-no fufu shusseiryoku hendo to sono kitei yoin (Changes in marital fertility and their determinants in Japan) (in Japanese). *Jinko Mondai Kenkyu (Journal of Population Problems)* 54(4): 3–18.

Screech, Timon. 2005. *Japan Entolled and Deciried: Carl Peter Thunberg and the Shogun's Realm, 1775–1796*. London: Routledge.

Sechiyama, Kaku. 1996. *Higashi Asia-no Kafuchosei: Gender-no Hikaku Shakaigaku* (in Japanese). Tokyo: Keiso Shobo.

Semba, Yukari. 2002. Funin to seishoku hojo gijutu-no genjo to kadai (Current status and problems of infertility and reproductive technology from a demographic perspective) (in Japanese). *Jinkogaku Kenkyu (The Journal of Population Studies)* 31: 37–46.

Shichijo, Tatsuhiro, and Mayumi Nishimoto. 2003. Wakai sedai-no fufu-no kodomosu-ni eikyo-wo oyobosu yoin (An analysis of factors that influence the number of children young married couples have in Japan) (in Japanese). *Riron to Hoho (Sociological Theory and Methods)* 18(2): 229–236.

Shigeno, Yukiko, and Katsumi Matsuura. 2003. Shussan, ikuji to shugyo-no ryoritsu-wo mezashite: kekkon, shugyo sentaku to kikon, shugyo josei-ni taisuru ikuji kyugyo seido-no koka-wo chushin-ni (Toward combining work and childbirth: Effect of parental leave on fertility of working married women) (in Japanese). *Kikan Shakai Hosho Kenkyu (The Quarterly of Social Security Research)* 39(1): 43–54.
Shirahase, Sawako. 2007. Women's economic status and fertility: Japan in cross-national perspective. In *Political Economy of Japan's Low Fertility,* ed. Frances McCall Rosenbluth, 37–59. Stanford: Stanford University Press.
Suruga, Terukazu, and Jian-Hua Chang. 2003. Ikuji kyugyo seido-ga josei-no shussan to keizoku shugyo-ni ataeru eikyo-ni tsuite (in Japanese). *Kikan Kakei Keizai Kenkyu (Japanese Journal of Research on Household Economics)* 59: 56–63.
Suruga, Terukazu, and Mayumi Nishimoto. 2002. Ikuji shiensaku-ga shussei kodo-ni ataeru eikyo (The effect of parental leave on childbirth) (in Japanese). *Kikan Shakai Hosho Kenkyu (The Quarterly of Social Security Research)* 37(4): 371–379.
Suzuki, Toru. 2001. Jinko gensho shakai-no shinzoku shigen (Kinship resources in declining population) (in Japanese). *Riron to Hoho (Sociological Theory and Methods)* 16(2): 185–197.
Suzuki, Toru. 2003. Rika-no doko, seisa, ketteiin (Leaving home in japan: Its trends, gender differences, and determinants) (in Japanese). *Jinko Mondai Kenkyu (Journal of Population Problems)* 59(4): 1–18.
Suzuki, Toru. 2005. Why is fertility in Korea lower than in Japan? *Jinko Mondai Kenkyu (Journal of Population Problems)* 61(4): 23–39.
Suzuki, Toru. 2008. Korea's strong familism and lowest-low fertility. *International Journal of Japanese Sociology* 17: 30–41.
Suzuki, Toru. 2011. Nikkan-no setai keisei pattern (Household formation behaviors in Japan and Korea) (in Japanese). *Jinko Mondai Kenkyu (Journal of Population Problems)* 67(3): 1–12.
Suzuki, Toru. 2006. Lowest-low fertility and governmental actions in Japan. The PIE International Conference on Declining Fertility in East and Southeast Asian Countries, Hitotsubashi Collaboration Center, Tokyo.
Tabuchi, Rokuro. 1998. Roshin-seijinshi dokyo-no kitei yoin: Kodomo-no seibetsu kosei-wo chushin-ni (Determinants of parent-adult child coresidence: The case of Japanese elderly women) (in Japanese). *Jinko Mondai Kenkyu (Journal of Population Problems)* 54(3): 3–19.
Tabuchi, Rokuro, and Hideki Nakazato. 2004. Roshin to seijinshi tono kyoju kankei: Dokyo, rinkyo, kinkyo, enkyo-wo megutte (in Japanese). In *Gendai Kazoku-no Kozo to Hen'yo: Zenkoku Kazoku Chosa (NFRJ98)-ni yoru Keiryo Bunseki (Structure and Change in Contemporary Japanese Families: Quantitative Analyses of National Family Research (NFRJ98))*, eds. Hideki Watanabe, Akihide Inaba, and Naoko Simazaki, 121–148. Tokyo: University of Tokyo Press.
Tanaka, Keiko. 2008. Jidoteate-no kakuju to kosodate setai-no kakei (in Japanese). *Kikan Kakei Keizai Kenkyu (Japanese Journal of Research on Household Economics)* 80: 39–44.
The Japan Institute for Labour Policy and Training (Dokuritsu Gyosei Hojin Rodo Seisaku Kenkyu-Kensyu Kiko). 2013. *Rodoryoku Juyo-no Suikei: Rodoryoku Jukyu Model (2012-nenban)-ni yoru Seisaku Simulation* (in Japanese). Shiryo Series No.110.
Todd, Emanuel, and Harumi Ishizak. 2001. *Sekaizo Kakumei* (in Japanese). Tokyo: Fujiwara Shoten.
Tsuya, Noriko O. 1999. Shusseiritsu teika to kosodate shien seisaku (Fertility decline and family policy in Japan) (in Japanese). *Kikan Shakai Hosho Kenkyu (The Quarterly of Social Security Research)* 34(4): 348–360.
Tsuya, Noriko O., and Linda G. Martin. 1992. Living arrangements of elderly Japanese and attitudes toward inheritance. *Journal of Gerontology* 47(2): S45–S54.
Tsuya, Noriko O., and Karen Oppenheim Mason. 1995. Changing gender roles and below-replacement fertility in Japan. In *Gender and Family Change in Industrial Countries*, eds. Karen Oppenheim Mason and AnMagritt Jensen, 139–167. Oxford: Clarendon Press.
Umezao, Tadao. 1957. *Bunmei-no Seitai Shikan* (in Japanese). Tokyo: Chuokoronsha.
United Nations Development program. 2013. *Human Development Report 2013.*

United Nations Population division. 2013. *World Population Prospects, 2012 Revision.*

van de Kaa, Dirk. 1987. Europe's second demographic transition. *Population Bulletin* 42(1): 1–59.

van Imhoff, Evert. 2001. On the impossibility of inferring cohort fertility measures from period fertility measures. *Demographic Research* 5(2): 24–64.

Vogel, Ezra F. 1991. *The Four Little Dragons*. Cambridge: Harvard University Press.

Wall, R. 1989. Leaving home and living alone: A historical perspective. *Population Studies* 43: 369–389.

World Economic Forum. 2012. *The Global Gender Gap Report 2012.*

Yamagami, Toshihiko. 1999. Shussan, ikuji to joshi shugyo tono ryoritsu kanosei-ni tsuite (Childbearing, childrearing and their compatibility with female labor supply) (in Japanese). *Kikan Shakai Hosho Kenkyu (The Quarterly of Social Security Research)* 35(1): 52–64.

Yamaguchi, Kazuo. 2005. Shoshika-no kettei yoin-ni tsuite: Otto-no yakuwari, shokuba-no yakuwari, seifu-no yakuwari (in Japanese). *Kikan Kakei Keizai Kenkyu (Japanese Journal of Research on Household Economics)* 66: 57–67.

Yang, Ching-Li, et al. 2012. Jin ershiniande guocheng jiegou bianqian (in Chinese). In *Taiwande Sahui Bianqian 1985–2005: Jiazu yu Hunyin*, ed. Academica Sinica, 1–28.

Yap Mui Teng. 2009. Ultra-low fertility in Singapore. In *Ultra-low Fertility in Pacific Asia,* eds. Gavin Jones, P. T. Straughan and Angelique Chan, 160–175. London: Routledge.

Yashiro, Naohiro. 2000. Shoshika mondai-heno keizaigakuteki approach (in Japanese). *Kikan Kakei Keizai Kenkyu (Japanese Journal of Research on Household Economics)* 4: 20–27.

Yashiro, Naohiro. 1999. *Shoshi Koreika-no Keizaigaku: Shijo Jushi-no Kozo Kaikaku* (in Japanese). Tokyo: Toyo Keizai.

Yuyama, Tomiko. 2006. Buyo to sen'yo: Chugoku-ni okeru fuyo system to oyakokan (in Japanese). In *Kazoku-no Hen'yo to Gender: Shoshi Koreika to Globalka-no Nakade*, eds. Takeshi Tomita and Lee Chong-Hwa, 239–268. Tokyo: Nihon Hyoronsha.

MIX
Papier aus verantwortungsvollen Quellen
Paper from responsible sources
FSC® C105338

If you have any concerns about our products,
you can contact us on
ProductSafety@springernature.com

In case Publisher is established outside the EU,
the EU authorized representative is:
Springer Nature Customer Service Center GmbH
Europaplatz 3, 69115 Heidelberg, Germany

Printed by Libri Plureos GmbH
in Hamburg, Germany